Praise for *Dieting with my Dog*

"*Peggy Frezon has written a charming and delightful tale.* Dieting with My Dog *is sweet, funny, inspiring and adorable, just like Peggy and Kelly!*" – Julie Klam, bestselling author of *You Had Me at Woof: How Dogs Taught Me the Secrets of Happiness*

"Dieting with My Dog *presents delightful incentives to improve health for people and their canine companions. With the book's rare combination of humor, practicality, and inspiration, readers will become motivated to lose weight and gain a special bond with their dog.*" – Linda Anderson, co-founder of Angel Animals Network, and co-author of *Dogs and the Women Who Love Them*, co-author of *Animals and the Kids Who Love Them*

"*It only took my reading the first page of Peggy Frezon's book,* Dieting with My Dog, *and I was hooked! As someone who has dealt with the challenges of weight gain and weight loss all of my life, I was inspired by Peggy's heart-warming story of her journey to make a positive change in her life with the help of her beloved dog, Kelly. Peggy blends humor, candor, and practicality in a wonderful way.*" – Julie Hadden, from NBC's 'The Biggest Loser' and author of *Fat Chance, Losing the Weight, Gaining My Worth*

"*A quirky and engaging tale of one woman's uncommon solution to a common problem. A moving and instructive celebration of the bond between humans and animals.*" – Ptolemy Tompkins, author of *The Divine Life of Animals*, former editor at *Guideposts* magazine.

"*Your dog relies on you to keep him healthy. This book is an excellent way to keep the both of you in nice shape; most importantly, by doing it together.*" – Joel Silverman, Host of Animal Planet's 'Good Dog U' and author of *What Color Is Your Dog?*

"*Everyone who has ridden the emotional rollercoaster of weight gain and loss, and struggled with the necessary lifestyle changes, will relate to Peggy's battle and eventual triumph over food's controlling grip. Her faithful dog is both an ally and a benefactor of the author's successful journey.*" – Dawn Kairns, author of *MAGGIE: The dog who changed my life*

"Dieting with My Dog *is the book I've been waiting for. This book will inspire you to get fit and love life as Peggy did – with heart, soul, and a best friend!*" – Nina Marinello, PhD, Nutrition Educator, Columnist – 'The Healthy Professor,' Albany (NY) Times Union. Coordinator of Sports Nutrition, Department of Athletics, University at Albany, State University of New York

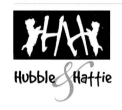
Hubble & Hattie

The Hubble & Hattie imprint was launched in 2009 and is named in memory of two very special Westies owned by Veloce's proprietors.
Since the first book, many more have been added to the list, all with the same underlying objective: to be of real benefit to the species they cover, at the same time promoting compassion, understanding and co-operation between all animals (including human ones!)
Hubble & Hattie is the home of a range of books that cover all-things animal, produced to the same high quality of content and presentation as our motoring books, and offering the same great value for money.

More titles from Hubble & Hattie

Animal Grief: How animals mourn each other (Alderton)
Cat Speak (Rauth-Widmann)
Clever dog! Life lessons from the world's most successful animal (O'Meara)
Complete Dog Massage Manual, The – Gentle Dog Care (Robertson)
Dieting with my dog (Frezon)
Dog Cookies (Schöps)
Dog Games – stimulating play to entertain your dog and you (Blenski)
Dog Speak (Blenski)
Emergency First Aid for dogs (Bucksch)
Exercising your puppy: a gentle & natural approach – Gentle Dog Care (Robertson & Pope)
Fun and Games for Cats (Seidl)
Know Your Dog – The guide to a beautiful relationship (Birmelin)
My dog is blind – but lives life to the full! (Horsky)
My dog is deaf – but lives life to the full! (Willms)
My dog has hip dysplasia – but lives life to the full! (Haüsler)
My dog has cruciate ligament injury – but lives life to the full! (Haüsler)
Older Dog, Living with an – Gentle Dog Care (Alderton & Hall)
Smellorama – nose games for dogs (Theby)
Swim to recovery: canine hydrotherapy healing – Gentle Dog Care (Wong)
Waggy Tails & Wheelchairs (Epp)
Walking the dog: motorway walks for drivers & dogs (Rees)
Winston ... the dog who changed my life (Klute)
You and Your Border Terrier – The Essential Guide (Alderton)
You and Your Cockapoo – The Essential Guide (Alderton)

www.hubbleandhattie.com

Cover photo: courtesy Ric Easton

First published in August 2011 by Veloce Publishing Limited, Veloce House, Parkway Farm Business Park, Middle Farm Way, Poundbury, Dorchester, Dorset, DT1 3AR, England. Fax 01305 250479/e-mail info@hubbleandhattie.com/web www.hubbleandhattie.com ISBN: 978-1-845844-06-6 UPC: 6-36847-04406-0.
Readers with ideas for books about animals, or animal-related topics, are invited to write to the editorial director of Veloce Publishing at the above address.
British Library Cataloguing in Publication Data – A catalogue record for this book is available from the British Library. Typesetting, design and page make-up all by Veloce Publishing Ltd on Apple Mac. Printed in India by Replika Press.

Visit Hubble and Hattie on the web: www.hubbleandhattie.com and www.hubbleandhattie.blogspot.com • Details of all books • Special offers • Newsletter • New book news

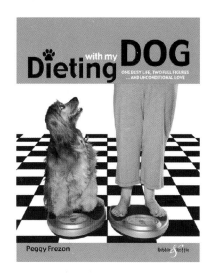

Peggy Frezon

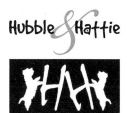

Acknowledgments

Thank you, Jude Brooks, for believing in a new author and her little dog. And to all the good folks at Hubble and Hattie.

So much love and thanks to my family: Mike, who loves and supports me totally. Kate and Andy, the reasons why the empty nest was so difficult – and so endurable. Mom, who instilled in me a love of all animals, especially the furry, tail-wagging ones who shared our home. Betty and Ed for their constant support. And, of course, to Kelly for being the best weight loss buddy ever.

Special thanks to Rick Hamlin, Edward Grinnan, Colleen Hughes, and everyone at Guideposts for teaching me how to shape the marble. To my critiquers: Sue Karas, Catherine Madera and Wanda Rosseland, and to the rest of the wonderful Marbleshapers: Stephanie Thompson, Julie Garmon, Mary Lou Reed, and B J Taylor. Also for your support: Judy Bastille, Alexis Grant, Shawnelle Eliasen, Aline Newman, Ginger Rue, Joy Choquette, Linda Shrake, and Dr Lisa Dietrich, DVM. To Jennifer May Photography, and to Ric Easton for photography and graphics editing skills. Also to Rebecca Nicholls of Eventageous PR.

Soli Deo Gloria.

Peggy Frezon
Rensselaer
New York

 Dedicated to Mike, who loves me through thick and thin

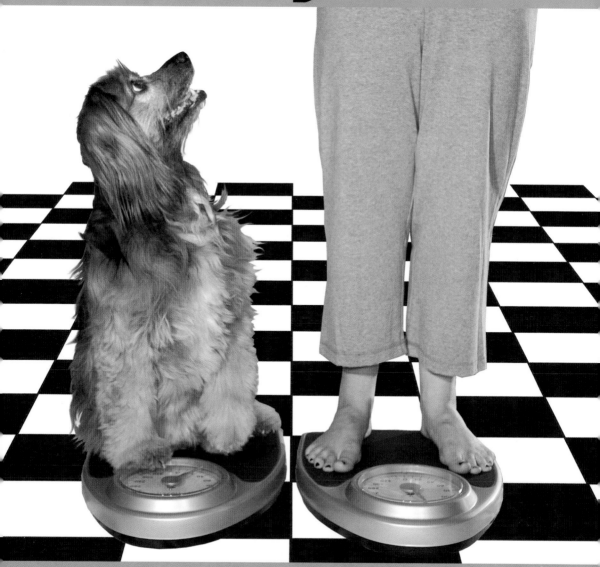

Dieting with my DOG

with my

ONE BUSY LIFE, TWO FULL FIGURES
... AND UNCONDITIONAL LOVE

Peggy Frezon

Hubble & Hattie

Contents

The tail end … … … … … … … … … … … … … … … … … …7

Puppy love … … … … … … … … … … … … … … … … … …8

Bone of contention … … … … … … … … … … … … … … .16

Basic obedience … … … … … … … … … … … … … … … .21

Chow down… … … … … … … … … … … … … … … … .27

Agility training .. … … … … … … … … … … … … … … .36

Old dog, new tricks… … … … … … … … … … … … … .48

Treats and retreats… … … … … … … … … … … … … .54

Wet nose, shiny coat. … … … … … … … … … … … … .62

Dog days of summer … … … … … … … … … … … … .66

A pat on the head.. … … … … … … … … … … … … .72

Dogcessories … … … … … … … … … … … … … … .77

Like chasing my tail .. … … … … … … … … … … … .85

The dog's dinner … … … … … … … … … … … … … .90

Every dog has her day.. … … … … … … … … … … … .94

It's a dog's life … … … … … … … … … … … … … … .99

Dog and dog parent weight loss tips from

    Peggy, Kelly and friends… … … … … … … … … … … 102

Diet notes .. … … … … … … … … … … … … … … … 112

The tail end

Let's face it: her butt was too big. Like many gals, she carried her weight in her hips. I glanced at Kelly sitting on the couch beside me, the late afternoon sun highlighting her silhouette. Her long, auburn hair fell softly on her shoulders. I didn't mean to cast a critical eye, but all at once it became clear. She was fat. Overweight. It wasn't fair to say obese, but certainly she'd packed on too many pounds. Too bad, I thought. She has such a pretty face.

Of course, who was I to talk? I freed the snap on the waistband of my jeans, expanding the breathing space mercifully. An image popped into my mind. Just a few months earlier I'd gone apple picking with my mom. There she was, walking ahead of me along a dusty country road, her backside as round as one of the rosy apples we were gathering. Far from being judgmental, I recognized a commonality. It could have been my own rear view. Mom and I are both short, with thick waists and ample curves. If we'd been dressed head to toe in scarlet, we might have appeared to have fallen directly from a Red Delicious tree!

I turned my attention again to Kelly lounging beside me on the living room sofa.

Sure, it stands to reason that family members sharing the same gene pool may eventually take on similar shapes. Only, the attractive redhead I was assessing beside me is not related. She barks up a different family tree altogether.

Kelly is not my mother or my daughter.

I was looking at my dog.

Puppy love

Kelly sprawled on the couch, a study in lethargy. Her little paws tucked under her chin, her eyes closed softly with that peaceful expression of total serenity. Long, shiny fur flowed around her body like a silken gown.

God, I wish I was a dog.

Maybe that thought crossed my mind more often than it should, but Kelly's life looked pretty good from where I was standing. Naps. Comfy beds. Delectable snacks tossed directly into her mouth whenever she looked hungry.

I, on the other hand, sat behind a Jenga tower of papers, attempting to create order atop my cluttered old computer desk. I worked from home, researching academic tests and writing for magazines and websites. Each weighty document demanded equal attention. Maybe they'd all tumble to the ground if I yanked the wrong one. Rubbing my temples, my head drooped toward the desk calendar, and thoughts of a nap sprang to mind. As I considered this, Kelly roused from the couch and crept over. I didn't know she was there until her gentle breath grazed my leg. She leaned against my desk chair and inched her chin onto my knee.

My husband and I had always shared our home with big dogs – ones that took up the length of the bed, or the entire couch. Kelly was the first lap-sized dog to join the family. And, with her long, swooping eyelashes and delicate features, the first girl dog. Even the way she crossed her paws under her chin when she slept suggested a dainty royal lady waiting to be served. Bring me my bone. Bring me my pink bunny toy. That's why it always takes me by surprise that – for all her self-centered and demanding behavior – Kelly also has an awareness, a presence of mind, that she can take care of me. When she jumps on the bed and smothers my face with furry kisses in the morning, it's as if she's encouraging me to start my day with a similar joyful energy. Or when she stops whatever she's doing and just looks at me, and in those stares something knowing passes between us, something deep and vulnerable and real.

I paused at my work. My hand slid across and rubbed Kelly's velvety head, sending waves of wellbeing to the tips of my fingers. I began to tap at the keyboard again.

I'd fallen for Kelly the moment I saw the pup with the bad hair day.

At that time our daughter, Kate, was a senior in high school and our son, Andy, was forging through his teen years. How could my kids be growing up so fast? How had those little ones, who had depended on me to get them dressed and tuck them in, turned into independent young adults?

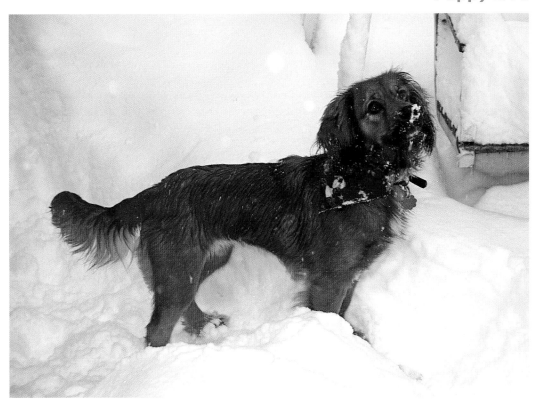

Kelly, about 9 months old, arrived from the rescue home in time to enjoy the new-fallen snow.

There had to be some way to stop the progression of time. Even our devoted Labrador Retriever was aging. Then an idea hit: a spry pup would be the perfect solution to the looming empty nest.

Searching for just the right dog on the rescue shelter website, face after furry, pleading face reached out to me, their hard luck stories making me ache to adopt them all. As I clicked on thumbnail photographs of countless small-to-medium-sized mixed breeds, however, I kept returning to Kelly. Her picture showed a gangly, seven- or eight month-old puppy with reddish fur – nearly the same shade as my kids' hair color. Crazy locks stuck out everywhere at improbable angles, forming a spiky mustache on her muzzle and giving her wild, wispy, brown eyebrows. An awkward cowlick rose from the back of her head. She was supposed to be a mix between Cocker Spaniel and some sort of smaller variety. Maybe a long-haired Dachshund. Who could tell? With mixed breed puppies, you could never be sure what you'd end up with.

It didn't matter. I wanted her.

"Do you think Hudson will get along with her?" Mike asked later, as we watched our potential new pet romp at the rescue home. Our sweet yellow Lab was twelve. In his younger days he'd tagged after the kids, chased tennis balls tirelessly, and splashed in the lake at my in-law's summer cabin. Lately, he'd slowed down, spending hours asleep with his big head resting on Mike's shoes.

"Maybe she'll help perk him up," I suggested.

Dieting with my dog

"Ya think?" Mike stared at the hyper pooch, whirling around like laundry in a spin cycle.

"Besides, it'll be nice to have a little one in the house again." I nudged Mike and grinned. "Easier than having another baby, right?"

He stepped back in surprise, clearly convinced I'd lost my mind.

When we brought Kelly home, the kids cradled her lovingly but Hudson barely lifted his head off the carpet. We placed the newcomer at his feet. She sniffed, pounced, then set off in search of more convincing life forms.

The main floor in our house is arranged in three boxy rooms. Dark, stained oak archways separate the hall from the living room, and another set stands between the living room and the dining room, where an open doorway leads into the kitchen, which connects back to the hall. Kelly lapped the circuit, as if being chased by a phantom greyhound. She bounced onto the sofa as if it were a trampoline, sprang into the dining room, then adeptly changed direction by ricocheting off a table leg.

"Something's wrong," I gasped.

"Is she hurt?" Mike asked.

"She doesn't seem to be."

"Well, maybe not physically, but …"

"Mentally?"

Then, just as suddenly as it began, the frenzy was over. Kelly collapsed on the rug, eyes closed and tongue lolling. A simple case of the 'puppy crazies.'

That year, my mind was spinning in circles, too. Kate was preparing to leave for college. Kate, who comfortably embraced me as confidante and respected me as parent. Kate, who told me about her first kiss and willingly friended me on Facebook. She actually liked to shop with me, and wasn't embarrassed if we ran into her classmates. I sat on the edge of her bed every night and listened as she expressed her hopes and shared her worries. While my friends complained that their daughters were secretive; shutting themselves behind bedroom doors, or drama queens; demanding the household's complete attention, I had Kate. I was blessed with this rare jewel of a relationship. I didn't want that to change; letting go of my daughter, my friend, meant giving up something I valued and wanted to keep close.

Kelly blended into our family easily, but of course that didn't stop the kids from growing up. She sat at my side as Andy borrowed the car keys, and hustled to and from basketball and baseball practices. She snuggled on the back of the couch, curling around my neck like a scarf, while I chatted with Kate on my cell phone. The nest didn't completely empty right away, as our happy family reunited when Kate returned for long winter breaks and summer vacations.

Then Kate graduated. Right out of college she married Aaron, a fellow graduate, and they blissfully began their life together in Virginia, more than 400 miles from our New York home. Yes, this was a natural progression into adulthood – and of course I took comfort in her success and happiness. But it felt like a long way for my mama wings to stretch.

At the same time Andy had become a high school senior, Hudson was gone, and Kelly had long since left the puppy crazies behind. Instead, mid-life Kelly lazily engaged in a sequence of naps, shifting between her favorite spots while I tapped at the computer nearby.

There was comfort in observing the uniformity of her day; watching her stretch out beside the bookshelf, knowing that next she'd move to her pillow in the corner, following her patterns while my keyboard emitted a pleasant, steady clicking. A crinkle of paper caught her attention for a moment, but then she put her head down again and snored, breaking the quietness that hung over the room. She rolled onto her side with exaggerated effort, her soft, white belly becoming visible, an iceberg in a sea of fur. Long, red and brown hair on her body usually hid her tummy, just like my baggy sweats camouflaged mine (I hoped). Or the stretchy, elastic waisted pants I wore that could e-x-p-a-n-d with me. And the shapeless tents that hung light and loose over bulges easy to deny if I didn't look. "What a pair," I told Kelly.

We were both overweight, no use pretending otherwise.

I'd tried dozens of diets. Every time a little weight managed to melt away, the pounds soon came back, and brought along a few friends, besides! After many years of on-again-off-again, my weight loss efforts felt like wading against the tide, and chances were I'd end up where I started.

My home 'office' consisted of a desk and a bookshelf tucked into a first floor corner of the house – only eight easy steps away from the kitchen. This was undeniably a favorable feature, as easy access to crunchy cookies eased the stress of demanding assignments. And who would deny that chocolate-covered candies and squares of creamy caramel made agreeable work companions?

After hours of researching and writing, thoughts of visiting these delicious officemates pushed productivity aside. Was it hunger that lured me away from my work and pulled Kelly away from her soft spot on the sofa? Or the idea of something, a little something, to fill an empty space? I slid back my chair and counted off the steps to the kitchen, Kelly at my heels.

Few needs ruled her life. The living room couch. A choice spot on my clean comforter. Full dinner bowls. An open door for trips in and out. Unlimited love and affection – happily provided, and equally returned. Our bond was evident whenever I left the house and Kelly waited at the front door, pressing her nose against the glass to watch for my return. As soon as my feet hit the porch and the door cracked open, she'd push past Mike, the kids, anyone who walked inside first, just to get to me, only me. She'd jump up, her front paws on my legs, and whimper, as if

being separated had been almost too much to bear. Despite this genuine adoration, however, another (greater?) love held sway in her heart. I believed with some certainty that she'd hurtle past my welcoming arms for a juicy hunk of steak.

We both paused at the refrigerator. Kelly parked herself at my feet, the tip of her tail thumping.

"What are you looking at?"

There was only one answer. Her wide, liquid brown eyes reflected the desperation of a half-starved stray on the street. Although her dinner bowl never stayed empty, that made little difference. Kelly knew the kitchen was a land of untold delicacies concealed in the chilly monolith her guardian stood before several times a day. Chances were a morsel would be shared, or just as likely dropped, making it fair game.

Sadly, a scan of the fridge revealed nothing tempting. The produce drawer sported onions, carrots, four limp stalks of celery, and a spongy orange. I bought fruits and veggies with the best of intentions: occasionally, I even ate some.

No tempting aromas filled my kitchen; baking proficiency was missing from my skill set. The pantry cupboard, however, held a cache of store-bought contentment: corn chips, cheese puffs, chocolate chip cookies. Propped up against a set of cobalt blue canisters bulged a bright cellophane bag: M&M's, my ruin.

A wonderful thrill washed over me, just like when I was a kid opening my treasured box of Crayola crayons, the colors delighting my imagination. Bright orange. Cheerful green. Dependable brown. M&M's came in colors for every occasion, too. I bought them all: bright reds and greens for Christmas; speckled Easter pastels; all pink for Breast Cancer Awareness month. Plain or peanut (and occasionally almond, mint, dark chocolate, raspberry or dulce de leche) it didn't matter – contrary to the classic slogan, I never gave my M&M's the opportunity to prove they would melt in my mouth, not in my hand.

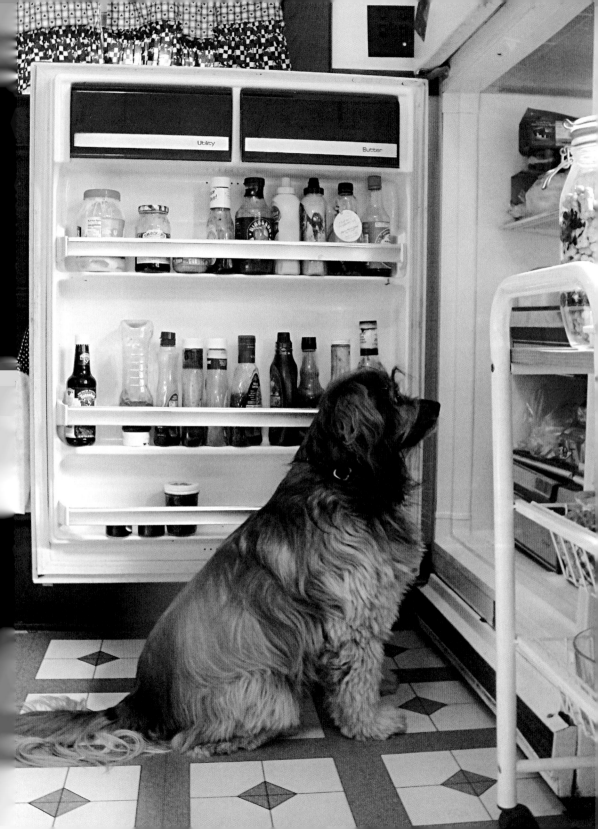

"Let's see, I'll have the burger meat, and the cheese … and, oh, gotta have some bacon!"

The bag seal parted easily. I downed a few candies, savoring their sweet, chocolatey smoothness. Kelly whined until I reached into the dog biscuit bin and tossed her a snack of her own. On such a dark winter afternoon, when fatigue settled in with the waning hours, we deserved a treat. Just one more. Who was I kidding? I sneaked my hand back into the M&M's bag.

A rap at the door startled me. Andy was still at school. Obviously, Mike didn't knock when he came home. Kelly's ears perked. Like a kid caught in the cookie jar, I scrambled to hide the evidence, shoving the candy bag behind the spaghetti canister. The bag tipped over, causing miniature colored gems to cascade to the floor. Although chocolates were my poison of choice, for dogs they actually are poison. Between kicking away the fallen chocolates so Kelly wouldn't devour them, and tripping over her as she wove between my feet, I looked like an inept tightrope walker from Cirque de Pathetique.

Another knock. Kelly barked and jumped. Peeking down the hall, I grabbed her webbed collar. "Shhhh!"

The purple stripe of the Federal Express deliveryman's sleeve flashed through the beveled panes in the front door. I tried to squeeze into the pantry corner to avoid being spotted. "Just leave the package and get out of here," I muttered under my breath.

Ordinarily, the FedEx guy didn't send me into a desperate search for a hiding place. But just look at me! A shapeless, nearly threadbare pink sweatshirt hung below my belly, over a bottom half crammed into my husband's old plaid flannel pajama pants. Blue fuzzy slippers completed this unusual ensemble. Not even a bra lurked underneath it all. I was definitely in no shape to hang out unsupported. No one should have to see that.

After one last knock, the purple stripe retreated. Kelly broke loose and ran to the front door, barking a message: "Wait, she's here, hiding in the pantry in her pajamas!"

"Thanks a lot," I muttered, slinking out of the corner, ruffling Kelly's ears nonetheless. While her facial hair was comically unruly, her long, silky ears resembled a schoolgirl's pigtails, and I liked to dress them up with ribbons the way I used to with Kate's long hair when she was a little girl. Kelly yawned, returned to the living room and reclaimed her napping spot. When I ambled toward the stairs, a direction that held less promise than the kitchen, she only stretched and shook her head.

Each step along the uphill climb to the second floor elicited a pitiful grunt. Old, lame dogs could move faster than I did. At 46, I had no excuse for being so out of shape. I was panting like a weary hiker. High blood pressure, high cholesterol – all those little pills in the compartmentalized box next to the salt and pepper shakers didn't lie. My body carried a good fifty pounds of excess weight, not that there was anything good about them. It used to be easy to explain away. Baby fat, as new moms liked to call it. Sweet, cute baby fat. Anyone can forgive the extra pounds put on after having a baby. But my children were far from babies. They were walking, talking, growing, going, driving, dating … and moving away. I stopped at the head of the stairs and peeked into Kate's empty room.

I clearly remembered the day I'd stood in Kate's college dorm room. "I'll call you every day," I'd said that muggy August afternoon as we watched her unpack. "I'll sit on the edge of your bed at home and we'll talk, like we've always done."

Dieting with my dog

"Of course." Kate pulled a whiteboard out of a canvas duffle bag and placed it on a shelf above her new desk.

"And pop a can of Diet Coke. You can have one, too, and we'll pretend we're drinking them together."

"Sure Mom," she said smiling gently, leaning over to give me a hug. But she couldn't hide the shift of her head, turning slightly toward the other freshmen in the hall passing by her open dorm door. Her attention focused ahead, mine still looking back.

That night, after we had made the long drive home from Cornell, I tiptoed into Kate's room and sat in the dark on the edge of her bed. The stillness pressed in tight. I raised my soda can to my lips and hit speed dial on my cell. After several lingering rings, I whispered to the voicemail recording, "Just Mom. We'll talk later."

Before long I'd found myself in the kitchen, in the dark, with a spoon and a carton of Fudge Ripple ice cream.

Although that was years ago, I still missed our face-to-face talks.

After resting a moment at the top of the stairs, I slipped into Kate's room. My hand glided across the soft, blue comforter on the neatly-made bed. After Kate left, Mike suggested transforming her room into an office. My home business was growing, and the move would de-clutter our living space, give me a serious, dedicated place to organize my work. Years later, though, everything was still the same. Although Kate wouldn't be coming home, I couldn't change that room.

I'd only encroached upon one space there, a tiny bit; Kate's vacant walk-in closet. Mike and I had always shared a small, cramped wardrobe space in our bedroom, so moving my clothes onto Kate's empty hanging rod made sense.

I opened the closet door. Bulky knits and over-sized shirts clothed the metal hangers where Kate's stylish tops and skirts used to hang. A spot of bright, autumn-orange peeked out of the row of blouses and sweaters. Last fall

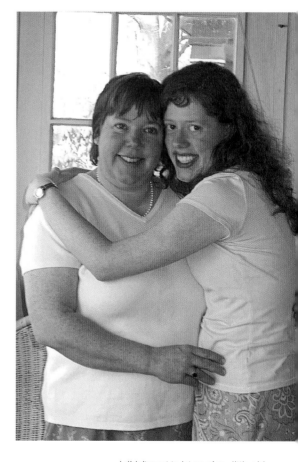

I didn't want to let go of my little girl.

I'd proudly purchased that orange fleece from a better quality women's store. A zipper ran up the front, and curved, black seaming embellished the sides. The latest tip from a fashion magazine suggested that these details were supposed to be slimming. Smiling in the mirror, I'd pulled on the jacket and went out to meet some friends.

Then, someone made a thoughtless comment. "You look like a basketball," she laughed lightly. She hadn't intended to be cruel, but just the same, my cheeks blazed with humiliation. I ran my hand along those 'slimming' seams, curving in a fine, full circle. How could I have imagined the top looked good?

I never wore that fleece again.

Below the fleece I'd stacked piles of bulging boxes full of smaller size clothing that hadn't been worn in years. I slid to the floor and slowly lifted a corner of one of the boxes. These clothes were no longer a part of my life. The old, slim me was gone. Kate was gone. And now Andy was preparing for college. In less than a year he would be moving out, too. My maternal duties were marked Done, Complete. I'd been let go after more than 18 years of service.

I prayed to God to stop all this, just return things to normal. After all, He could do anything. But the answer that came back to me was always the same; this is normal … this *is* normal.

Of course, the children's flights of independence were natural. Healthy, even. Great educations, new families, budding careers – all positives. But who would take care of them?

Would Kate's new husband know the way Kate's skin flushed across the bridge of her freckled nose when she started to get sick? Would Andy wear his sneakers with those crazy, no-show socks that left his ankles bare and defenseless when traipsing on campus in mountainous snow drifts?

And – where did all this leave me?

Huddling in the dark, the closet closed around me like a cocoon. Gradually, a warmth grew beside me, a gentle heat that blanketed my leg, extended to my waist and embraced my body. My hand reached out and touched Kelly's soft fur. She'd found me, quietly padded into the closet, and slipped in beside me. I stroked her back. Her sides moved as she breathed in and out. Slowly, rhythmically. She made tiny sighs. We stayed there for a long time, together.

Just breathing.

Bone of contention

I shrugged out of my cardigan and kicked off my shoes while the nurse waited. *Every little bit helps.* I stepped onto the scales. The nurse slid the weights in increments to the right ... *clack, clack, clack.* Then she scribbled an impossible-to-believe number on my chart.

For quite some time I'd refused to weigh myself at home. My clothes were straining at the seams and pinching at the waist. I didn't want to know more. But right there was the cold truth in black and white: 171 pounds. *Ugh.* That much weight was probably too much even for a six foot (maybe seven foot!) tall woman. It sure wasn't cute on my measly five foot frame.

In the examining room, the doctor fastened a blood pressure cuff around my arm. As it tightened, my anxiety increased, providing no benefit for my heart rate.

"Your blood pressure is not where we want it," he said, jotting down numbers. "What are you taking, one pill a day, right?"

I nodded.

"I think it's time to up your dosage."

Up my dosage? When first prescribed, the blood pressure medication seemed unnecessary. I didn't feel sick, and I certainly didn't want to start on some medication that I'd have to take for the rest of my life.

Now, the doctor was scribbling a new prescription for an even greater amount. His finger glided across a page as he read from my chart: "You've already got high blood pressure. And high cholesterol."

I nodded.

"Your labs indicate impaired glucose metabolism, which is a strong precursor to diabetes. And you have family history. Your father died of a heart attack when he was, um, 55 ... right?"

I nodded again.

Putting aside my folder, the doctor looked straight at me and frowned. "With your weight right now, you're high risk for some serious problems. Osteoporosis, arthritis, respiratory deficiencies, stroke, diabetes, heart disease, cancer, heart attack ..."

I squirmed on the examining table. Hadn't he mentioned the same at my last physical? I'd promised then to watch what I ate. And I had, for a little while. Then I slid back into my old habits.

"How much exercise do you get?" he asked.

"Umm, a little?" No use trying to fool the doctor. It was obvious I was no gym rat.

"You should walk, do aerobics, something, at least three days a week."

"I'll try." I said. And I really wanted to. I knew I should. But somehow, a few days later, I wasn't thinking about my doctor appointment anymore. I wasn't thinking about changing and getting sweaty and eating lettuce. I just went back to my busy routine at home, spending time with Mike and Andy, working, and taking care of Kelly.

Something was missing from my plate on the coffee table.

I returned from the kitchen with a can of diet cola to go with my golden grilled cheese, but only half a sandwich and a few telltale crumbs remained. Kelly sat directly in front of the scene, licking her lips, the picture of guilt.

"What'd you do?" I asked, drawing out the 'ooo' sound, my voice singing. Kelly's tail thwacked.

"You call that a scolding?" Mike asked, shaking his head.

"Kind of a scolding," I replied.

"I've seen firmer corrections from my grandmother," he teased.

"Well, she didn't *mean* to do it."

"What do you mean, she didn't mean to?" Mike moved the plate to higher ground. "Did someone force her to eat it? You've got to tell her *No!*"

He got me. Guilty. This wasn't the first time Kelly had snitched food off the table and I'd ignored it. I knew I shouldn't let her get away with this behavior. But when she looked at me with her big, innocent eyes and her tail wagging hopefully, I wanted to give her the other half of the sandwich as well. Instead, I scooped her an extra helping of dog food. Her bowl was empty, so she must have been hungry.

After lunch, I checked the clock and pulled on my coat. "Time to go!" Hearing this, Kelly sprang into action.

Mike jingled the car keys in his pocket and she danced around him. "It's not what you think, you big goof," he said.

I took the leash off the hook and clipped it to her collar. Kelly understood that the leash meant she was going out, and the keys meant a ride in the van. Sometimes, we headed to the park or the lake or somewhere fun. But she always forgot that sometimes the destination was someplace not so pleasant – the veterinarian's office.

She trotted along beside me as we left the house and jumped eagerly into the van, bouncing onto the long bench seat in the back as I slid into my own seat in the front. Before the van left the driveway, however, she'd squeezed over the console and bullied her way onto my lap. No matter how many times we put her in the back, the prime real estate of the front seat was always her objective. She stretched across my leg and pressed her nose to the window, breathing steamy smudges.

Once we stopped at the cedar-sided building outside of town, she tumbled eagerly out of the van and into the parking lot, still clueless of our location. Her tail wound in a rapid circle at the intoxicating variety of odors. At the walkway, however, she stopped short, recognizing something familiar – perhaps a little sinister – about this place. If not the shots and blood samples, a dog would scarcely forget various intimate examinations.

She balked as we approached the front door. "Awww. You don't want to go in." I sighed and tugged her toward the entrance. "Can't blame you. I don't like visiting the doctor's office either."

No wonder my dog and I got along so well during the day. Our wills most often aligned. She approved of sleeping in late and saw no point in hanging around outside for fresh air if the weather was cold or wet. We both knew the value of a warm snuggle and an afternoon snack. And we both preferred to avoid unpleasant encounters, such as doctor appointments.

Nevertheless, I urged Kelly inside. The waiting room only increased her anxiety as she realized all those tantalizing smells from outside belonged to a contingent of canines inside. The other dogs at once excited and frightened her. She alternated between pulling until she choked and cowering under Mike's seat. I smiled sheepishly at the other pet parents seated around the room.

The receptionist called our name at last and we started toward the examining room. Kelly

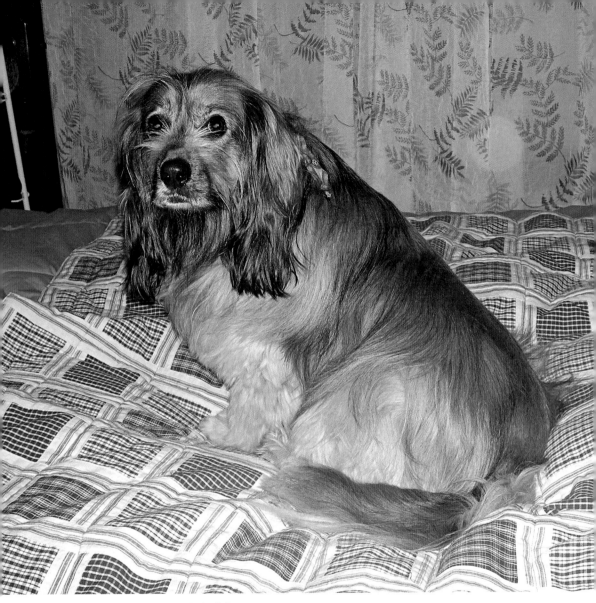

Extra pounds meant extra health risks for Kelly.

grabbed the leash in her mouth and tried to pull us in the opposite direction, out the door.

"Isn't she cute," the bubbly tech assistant said.

"Sure," Mike groaned.

When the doctor entered the tiny room she bent low and gushed, "Oh, here's a beautiful little girl, what a good girl."

Kelly instantly stopped panicking and sat beguilingly, her long-term memory failing her. Amazingly, the vet was able to win over the most manic mutt with just a little schmoozing.

"Let's see what we've got, here. *Ooof.*"

Dr Dietrich's eyes widened as she hefted Kelly onto the steel table.

Okay, so our gal wasn't a Chihuahua, but she was no Great Dane either!

After the mandatory pokes and prods, the

doctor lifted Kelly down. "Well, everything looks okay. Let's just get her weight."

There it was, the moment every girl dreaded. Kelly wasn't skinny, I accepted that. At the last few appointments the vet had suggested that Kelly weighed a bit more than she should. I'd nodded, but I never took it seriously. Kelly was fine. I'd never let her be in pain, or neglect to give her medication. Filling up her dog bowl was just filling her up with love.

Kelly followed our lead to an enormous floor scale and stepped up onto the rubber platform. Numbers on the digital readout bounced up and down as she wiggled.

"Stay still," I said, wishing I had a liver treat for bribery. Then I remembered why she was on the scale.

The doctor waited, and then scribbled on her record sheet. "Forty-one," she said.

I nodded and we prepared to leave.

This time, however, the vet shook her head. "She's up three pounds."

Well, perhaps the scales were off – scales were known to lie: mine at home did, all the time, recording numbers that couldn't possibly add up to the couple of extra treats I'd consumed during the day. The same for Kelly.

"And, remember, she was up a few pounds at her last visit, too," Dr Dietrich continued.

"She doesn't really overeat," I assured. "Only one scoop."

The doctor reached into a cupboard and held out a tiny plastic cup. "About this much?" she asked. Mike and I exchanged a guilty glance. The cup looked like a thimble compared to Kelly's scoop of dog food. "Half a cup, twice a day," the vet added. "And no table scraps."

Mike shot me a look.

As Kelly stood at the door, I took stock. Pot belly. Love handles. Wide rear end. All of a gal's most dreaded figure flaws, poor thing. It was just a matter of time and she'd look as heavy as Hudson in his later years.

Our beautiful yellow lab had once been sleek and muscular, but then grew far heavier. His sides bulged, his tummy sagged, and his neck hung with rolls of fat.

"Excess weight can lead to some serious health problems." The vet rubbed Kelly's sides for emphasis.

A chill went through my body.

Hudson hadn't just been fat. His health had suffered. Joint conditions made walking difficult. He panted excessively. His coat was lumpy; an orange-sized cyst bulged under his fur.

One sweltering afternoon I'd straddled his girth in the kitchen, trying to lift him. He was heavy and weak, and wet. He'd lost his continence. I wrapped my arms around his belly to help ease him to his feet. As we shuffled to the back door, he stumbled down the steps to the soft grass below. He could move, but his awkward gait told me each step was painful.

That night I'd knelt quietly beside him. He was sleeping, his paws twitching. We used to say, when he was younger, that he was dreaming about chasing rabbits. Now maybe he was just in pain. I didn't want him to suffer. Mike came and stood quietly beside us.

Hudson was well-loved – and well-fed.

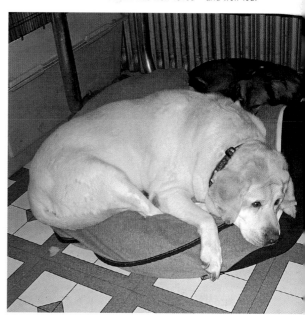

Dieting with my dog

"How will we know?" I'd asked him.

"He'll tell us."

Less than a week later we sat solemnly on the vet's cold examining room floor, flanking Hudson's yellow body. His tail beat a rhythm on the tiles. His big brown eyes stared up at us in trust. The vet held a syringe. "How can we allow this?" I thought.

We stroked Hudson's head, neck, his back. "You're a good boy," Mike said.

"I love you," I whispered. Hudson raised his head off my lap and licked my hand. Mike's eyes brimmed.

"Ready?" the vet had asked.

We hadn't responded.

"Ready?" Dr Dietrich asked now, after completing Kelly's examination. I pulled my thoughts away from that somber appointment several years ago, to Kelly's present predicament. She stood at the door, her plump body waggling as she waited. I wiped my eyes and thought of how painful it had been to lose Hudson. *What if it had been my fault?* How could I not have seen that the way I ate, my lack of exercise, had contributed to Hudson's escalating weight? If only I'd been able to help him shed some of those pounds, maybe I could have added some years to his life.

"Even a few pounds are a lot for a little dog,"

Dr Dietrich continued. "They could add up to more than 10 per cent of her body weight." The vet rubbed Kelly's sides for emphasis. "If she doesn't start losing weight, this could lead to bone and joint problems. Difficulty breathing. Increased blood pressure. Decreased energy and lack of stamina. Heart failure. There's a risk of diabetes, even cancer."

I swallowed hard. Those were real health issues. Not only that, but real health issues *I'd* heard before.

As the veterinarian stroked Kelly's fur and rattled off the same possible consequences of being overweight as my doctor had given me, I knew this was serious. I looked down at myself, then back at my chubby dog. We both weighed too much. We weren't just talking about heavy hips any more; we faced potential health risks – serious medical concerns – as a result of being fat. Despite haphazard attempts, there was no denying it. I wasn't really taking good care of myself, and it wasn't only me I was harming. My bad habits also hurt Kelly.

She pawed the examining room door. I couldn't deny the obvious. We were fat, and it was time to change. I stooped and hugged her neck. "We're going to lose some weight," I promised. "Together."

Basic obedience

Saturday night, and I sure knew how to live. While others enjoyed evenings at the movies or bars, or even at home in their own comfortable reclining chair, I was being dragged along sticky black rubber mats in a cavernous, industrially-tiled room. The local elementary school cafeteria had surely seen its share of chaos, but doggy obedience classes must have ranked right up there with Jell-O slinging and stomach ache.

I stopped to rest by a gray laminate table folded against the wall, a lingering whiff of Tater Tots mingling with a distinctively doggy odor. On the menu: one hour of basic canine training served with a scoop of humility.

Kelly added her own brand of fun to the proceedings, pulling at her leash with surprising strength for a pooch who could barely muster the energy to climb out of her cushy dog bed that afternoon. But it was time for Kelly to learn some manners.

"Stand with your dog at your side," began the instructor, as her model Golden Retriever moved into position, obeying a command so subtle I hadn't even noticed it myself.

Ten different dogs – barrel-chested, curly, sleek, kinky-tailed – fell into place at the left of their humans.

Kelly sat squarely in front of me, looking up.

"The *left* side," the instructor called pointedly in my direction.

I tugged the leash. Kelly lay down.

"Heh," I mumbled to a petite older woman handling what looked to be a mix between a German Shepherd and a cow. I felt my cheeks flaming. "She's just a little, uh, confused."

The woman flashed me one of those 'I'm just humoring you' smiles.

"Okay, class." The instructor's voice reverberated across the cafeteria. "Forward!" Her handsome Retriever (who I'd silently dubbed Captain Perfect) led the way. The first dog in line, a spunky terrier, trotted at the end of the leash held by his proud companion. One by one the dogs executed 'forward' as instructed. Kelly, lying at my feet, apparently had no intention of obeying. I took a hopeful step forward, focused on the rubber runners lining the path. Dogs and pet parents sidestepped, tripped, and collided into our back end as my dog refused to shift out of park.

I could swear Captain Perfect sneered at us when the class ended and we beat a hasty retreat. I felt like the unpopular kid in middle school who'd just dropped her lunch tray.

"How was obedience class?" Mike asked when we returned from our lesson. Kelly trotted to the kitchen and blissfully dug into her well-deserved dinner.

Dieting with my dog

"Kelly's not big on obedience," I said dryly. "That bad?"

"Well, there were twin Yorkies that yapped so much the instructor had to spray them with water. A Labradoodle that attempted a romantic liaison with a Beagle. One dog broke free and raced down the hall to the janitor's closet. Two dogs peed on the floor. And Kelly was still the worst one there."

"Guess she has some things to learn," Mike said.

"I guess." I absently grabbed a handful of M&M's from the pantry. Despite my efforts, Kelly had a knack for ignoring the simplest directions. She knew the recall command, but responded only when she wanted to. More often, she ran extra laps in the back yard when I called her in, which led to my shameful practice of tempting her inside with a biscuit. I knew better. What mom didn't know that bribing good behavior with food was a recipe for obesity? Still, a distorted recording played in my mind: she *deserved* that treat.

I returned to the living room, where Kelly sprawled across my favorite place on the couch. I crammed myself into the corner by the arm.

"Why don't you tell her to get down?" Mike asked.

I shrugged. Didn't she deserve a nice comfy spot on the couch, too? Why sacrifice her comfort for mine?

Mike shook his head at Kelly lounging contentedly while I scrunched up like a pretzel. "She's got it made," he said.

I guess he was right. Other pet parents had rules about dogs getting up on the furniture. Maybe I needed to be more firm. But why change something that did, in a way, work for me, too? I had to confess, she was nice and warm by my side.

Was I so unwilling to make adjustments in other areas of my life? Clearly, our kids kept growing and changing. What had started it all? Their first steps, when they no longer needed me for actual physical support to keep them

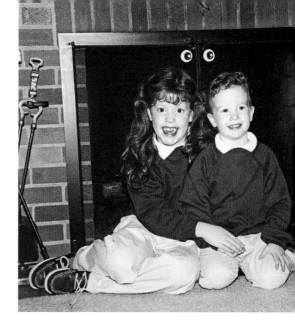

Kate and Andy (ages 7 and 3), when they still needed me for everything.

upright? When they could decide on their own whether they would totter into the safe living room, or attempt to climb the dangerous stairs; whether to stay on the sidewalk or suddenly jump into a tempting puddle, or even dart into the street? They kept maturing, separating, and it was up to me to adapt to this.

Now I had to accept more changes. The vet told me to modify Kelly's lifestyle. My doctor wanted me to eat differently and get healthy. I'd promised to start dieting, but I didn't even know where to begin.

I cringed, considering all the weight loss programs in my arsenal. The Cabbage Soup Diet. The Grapefruit Diet. The Green Tea Diet. And my personal favorite, the 7 Day, All You Can Eat Diet. *What's not to love about that one?* I even attempted sensible slimming programs like Weight Watchers. The trouble is, you actually have to stick to the diets for them to work. Yeah, right ...

Fewer calories. More fruits and veggies. I knew that stuff. No one gained weight because they actually thought cookies were healthier than carrots. Knowledge wasn't the problem. It was follow-through. There was no question that, in most cases, eating fewer calories and increasing physical activity resulted in weight loss. Yet, for years I'd moaned and complained that it was impossible to lose the flab. I'd searched for the magic solution that would make it all happen, when really it required just one step: obedience.

"Where to start?" I typed into a conversation on the Instant Messenger the next afternoon. Kelly pawed at my elbow, like a child begging for Mom's attention while she was on the phone. I got up, found a chewy snack and flipped it into the air. Although Kelly could devour this treat quicker than an ice cream melting on a hot summer day, I hoped she'd stay occupied long enough for a short chat.

More than anything, I hoped my friend, Judy, had figured out the secret key to weight loss. In fact, Judy was more than a friend, she was also my cousin. She had a son and a daughter a little older than Kate and Andy, and in many ways we were comfortably alike. Although she lived out of state and we didn't get to see each other often, we'd bonded long distance over our repeated failed diets. Every so often we made the same resolution to eat better and exercise, and for a time it worked.

A few years earlier I'd lost twenty-two pounds, while at the same time Judy 'found' a comparable amount. Now, as my waistline expanded, bulging out of a 16 dress size, heading relentlessly toward an 18, Judy was faithfully walking, watching what she ate, and shedding pounds.

"I dunno, we just have to start," Judy shot back. "Not easy when we're feeling fat and disgusting."

"True," I replied. "Hard to love thunder thighs and arm jiggle."

"Here's what I'm doing. I'm just trying to eat healthier now. You know better than anyone,

I've tried nearly every regimen out there. Even those weight loss pills my doctor prescribed, remember? But I decided I'm not going on another diet. This is more like a healthy eating plan. Sounds better, doesn't it?"

"I guess." It didn't really matter what you called it; when you couldn't eat what you wanted, it still amounted to that four-letter word. DIET. I adjusted a pillow behind my back and leaned over the keyboard.

"Whatever you're doing, I hope it helps."

I hated to admit it but I didn't have high hopes for my cousin. The Judy I knew liked to stop by the McDonald's drive-through for McCalories on her way home from church. She used her exercise bike as a clothes drying rack. The Judy I knew was just like me. We were sometimes on different pages, but we always arrived together at the end of the chapter.

"Seriously," I added, "I have all the reasons in the world to lose weight, but I can't seem to get going. You know when you look at yourself in a photograph, and you can't stand to look at it because your clothes hang over you like some sort of lawn furniture covering, and your face is so bloated and your body so distorted you don't even look like yourself anymore? But instead of changing my eating habits, I just stopped looking."

There was a pause before Judy responded. "I noticed my reflection in the pizza shop window, and that's when it hit for me. There has to be a moment, I guess. A moment so big that you know you have to change, right then and there. No more excuses."

"True. We can know *what* to do; we just have to obey and do it. A lot like Kelly." I told her about the debacle in the elementary school cafeteria.

"Keep trying," she returned. "Kelly will catch on. You just have to help her see it's for the best."

"I will," I replied. "And you keep it up too, okay?" I added, "Don't forget, strawberry Pop-Tarts are healthy. Fruit, right?"

Dieting with my dog

"Absolutely," Judy replied, with a little smiley face icon. "And gummy fish are seafood."

The next day, I sat at the dining room table, armed with paper, pen, and a stack of books; recipes, nutrition, self-help. It seemed like I had a million. Leafing through the pages, I waited for the magic words to leap out at me, the inspiration and motivation I'd been missing; the switch that would start the journey. I rubbed my eyes. My temples throbbed. But there was nothing new. Just hard work, low-fat food, exercise. I still hoped for a plan that involved hefty portions of ice cream. Maybe on the internet ...?

Switching to my computer desk in the corner, I opened my search engine and tapped in 'ice cream diet.' Result! My spirits soared as I clicked on the heading. This was it, the diet of my dreams. I imagined mounds of luscious fudge swirl, chocolate chip, and the 'health-conscious' strawberry (fruit). Heck, I'd even settle for plain vanilla, as long as it was ice cream.

But scrolling down the page, my dreams were dashed. The daily menu consisted of black coffee, some dry toast, a cup of plain tuna, string beans and only half a cup of low-fat ice cream. I sputtered in disgust.

Searching for more realistic options, I discovered 220 million hits for 'diet,' 180 million hits for 'exercise,' and more than 7 million for 'secret to weight loss.' Obviously, a hot topic. I clicked on the first few entries.

By the time Mike arrived home from work that night, I'd amassed an impressive pile of colored papers, computer printouts, and heavily highlighted charts. Books and magazines littered the dining table. Rulers, markers of every color, fancy paper clips, and even an over-enthusiastic chunk of poster board left over from one of the kids' science fair projects cluttered my work space.

"What are you up to?" Mike asked, loosening his tie as he walked into the room.

"Making our diet."

"*Ours?*" he asked.

"Sure. You're going to want to eat the same foods as me, right?"

He surveyed the papers. "Looks complicated."

"Not really." I held up a color-coded graph. "This tracks our weight, calories, different foods with points assigned to each ..."

"Yeah. Complicated."

Ignoring this, I held up another sheet. "And this one lists our unlimited options, yellow for proteins, green for veggies, blue for low-fat foods." He'd never believe how much time I spent on those plans. I wrote them over dozens of times, made posters, transferred data to spreadsheets on the computer. I collected recipes, categorized them, made grocery lists. "Oh, and here's a chart for restricted foods, and ..." I noticed Mike grinning. "I'm not joking around, you know."

"I can see that," he said. "So, what's for dinner?"

I looked from the charts in my hand to the pile of books. "Oh." The papers fluttered to the tabletop. "I hadn't thought about that."

For the first few days I followed my new plan with gusto. I carefully measured a serving of breakfast cereal each morning and prepared celery and carrots for my snacks. I marked everything down on my charts. Several days later, however, I realized some spaces were left blank. The next week even more blank spots filled the pages. I neatly stacked my diet books, from widest to smallest, and set them aside.

When we went out to the grocery store,

Kelly and I at our heaviest.

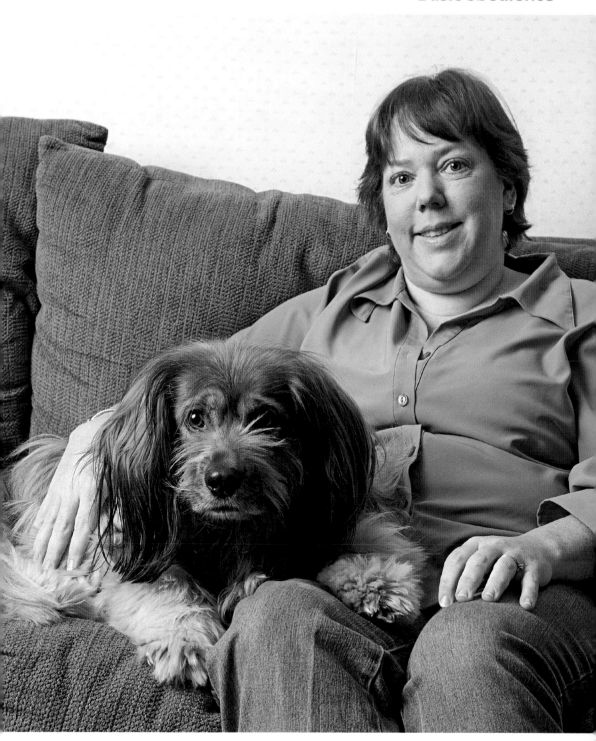

Dieting with my dog

I found myself ill-prepared. "What do we need for one of your new recipes?" Mike asked.

"I, uh, don't remember. The list is at home." Since we were in the produce section, I selected a bag of carrots and some rosy red apples. But a few aisles later, the contents of our cart regressed, with chips, pasta mixes and double-stuffed cookies covering up the meager healthy options on the bottom. It's like those foods just jumped into the cart of their own volition. Seriously.

Later, after stocking the fridge and cupboards, I lifted the corner of the pile of charts, peeking at the detailed plans. While creating the papers had been fulfilling, that's where the fun left off. I pushed them aside. Looking made it too real.

I'd ignored other problems in the past. I'd denied my jeans were too tight, neglected to take my blood pressure pills regulary. So I should have expected what came next. That familiar, heavy feeling of guilt. It pressed around me as I huffed my way up the stairs. It needled me when I reached for that bowl of ice cream before bed. Still, no checkmark of progress marred my perfectly penned posters. My Guilt-O-Meter climbed another notch.

It wasn't until one night when I was snuggled on the couch next to Kelly, relaxing after dinner, that the urgency sunk in. I was looking at a magazine, and Mike was reading his newspapers, when my cell phone rang.

"Sorry I haven't been in touch lately," said the voice on the other end. What a treat! My cousin, Judy, usually Instant Messaged me. We rarely talked on the phone. I guessed she was feeling bad that she'd been too busy to get on the computer.

But I gasped as she told me the real reason why she had called. "I've been in the hospital," she said.

"No, Judy! What happened? Are you okay?" My throat went dry as I mouthed the words to Mike across the room: "Heart attack." He raised his eyebrows.

"I'm home now, I'm doing better. I don't know, Peggy. I was just walking up the hill with my friends, we've been doing that after work, you know. I was kind of dragging, I thought I was just tired, with the time change and all. But then I felt this pressure, like an elephant sitting on my chest. It didn't hurt, exactly, but I knew something was wrong. I went to the ER and the next thing I knew, they were loading me into an ambulance, taking me to the cardiac care hospital."

I couldn't believe it. "You sure you're okay?"

After Judy filled me in on more details, I couldn't help blurting, "But I thought you were doing better. You were losing weight and everything."

"I was," she said. "But too late. Those bad habits had already done their damage. I'm actually lucky. The doctors took care of the blockage, and I'm going to be better than before."

I hung up the phone, worried. This was serious. Nervous tingles prickled my mind with a new thought. Judy's father and my dad were brothers. My dad had died of a heart attack at a young age. I already had a genetic risk factor. Maybe Judy and I shared hereditary traits that increased my odds for a heart attack, too. Maybe more importantly, we shared the same lifestyle. We both loved junk food and our sedentary habits. If Judy had a heart attack, it could happen to me. I thought of Mike and the kids; I had to stay healthy for them. Then I looked at Kelly, remembering our visit to the vet. What would happen to her if something happened to me? Kelly didn't deserve a companion who would give her treats. She deserved a friend who would be healthy and keep her healthy, too.

I didn't need fancy charts and tables. It was time for obedience.

The switch had flicked on.

Chow down

I'd fallen into the habit every evening of having a little snack before bed, then feeling ashamed for overeating. I'd followed this routine like following the instructions on a shampoo bottle: use liberally to maximize fullness. Rub (stomach thoroughly to soothe sick, overeating feeling). Rinse (away guilt by vowing to change the next day). Repeat.

Saturday morning, before even setting my feet on the floor, I made myself a promise: *today, there would be no 'Repeat.'*

The alarm went off. Kelly bounced onto the bed, burrowed her cold nose under the covers and poked me in the ribs. Although she was always eager to start the day, I needed a little more transition time.

"Gotta get moving or we'll be late," Mike said, shaking my shoulder. Kelly licked my closed eyelids; there went my transition time.

We were scheduled to take Andy to a program for accepted students at a university in the central part of New York, a three-hour drive. Although Andy had applied to colleges out of state, ones requiring a plane ride or an entire day's travel, ones that were farther than where Kate now lived – even this one, a manageable jaunt up the expressway, seemed too far away to me. I was excited for Andy, though, with all the promise and possibilities of college ahead of him.

Ideally, we should have started the day with a wholesome breakfast, but we only had time for toast. I pulled on my khakis and a sweater, and stuffed a few supplies into a bag to take along.

Andy moved uncharacteristically quickly to get ready to roll that morning. When he emerged from his room in loose jeans and a team t-shirt, I pictured a curly-haired baby boy in OshKosh overalls instead. He turned down some toast and sighed, leaning against the arm of a chair as Mike and I finished eating. While baseball season kept him busy, everything else became tedious and confining, and the inability to focus on anything – a classic case of Senioritis – made the last few months drag by for him. Accepted Student Day was his reminder that he actually had made progress.

I paused at the front door. "Be good," I told Kelly. My in-laws were coming to let her out – twice – but nevertheless Kelly's jumping for her leash, begging to come along, filled me with guilt. She wove between my legs to avoid being overlooked. I went to the kitchen and found her a biscuit. The treat would make her feel better while we left her alone. "We'll be back, don't worry."

"Peg …" Mike rolled his eyes. Who could blame him? Kelly whined. Before I could react, Mike took my arm. "She'll be fine," he said and elbowed me out the door.

We arrived at the university amid snarling traffic and clusters of families following

Dieting with my dog

backwards-walking student guides. Leave it to college students to multi-task; walking backwards, yet moving forward, while at the same time giving informative campus tours to prospective freshmen.

I'd once been great at juggling my job, children, school, and afternoon activities, all while getting a decent meal on the table. Not so much anymore. "I can barely keep up with her, and I'm walking forward," I puffed to Mike as we joined the group.

While Andy took in the guide's rundown on classes and social life, I studied the tall, gray stone library, each story rising higher, progressing like the years. I didn't picture Andy in this place, but only imagined our home without him.

Four-and-a-half years earlier I had experienced the same restless feelings as Kate took her first eager steps of independence. The anxious expressions of the parents on Andy's college tour were much like those of the moms and dads at Kate's freshman orientation. Back then, the Cornell University president had spoken to the group assembled on hard metal chairs in the stifling gymnasium.

"The challenge now," he had said, "is to watch your children fully experience this, to navigate the challenges before them, even to make mistakes.

"And to give up the idea that you can prevent those mistakes. The sense that you can protect them." It seemed like the president directed his next statement right at me. "Remember," he said, "they're ready for this."

Maybe so, but was I? I'd sniffed and looked away.

Now I was about to go through the same thing again. The tour group paused in front of the imposing, domed athletic stadium. Andy stood dazzled, thoroughly scanning the structure from ground to roof. If the exciting majors and attractive girls in skimpy summer tops hadn't yet convinced him, the gleaming, modern sports facility iced the cake.

The culminating event of the day was a series of open panel discussions over a buffet lunch. The school did its best to impress, and, ordinarily, I'd welcome such a spread. Long tables cloaked in white linen brimmed with crusty bread, orange squares of cheese stacked in tempting towers, deli meats with creamy dressings. And at the end, the reward; decadent bars of rich brownies and cookies in endless supply. I stopped short, remembering: I'd vowed to start eating sensibly.

We filed in line into the packed stadium, the buffet a walk of torture. My sandwich options were a golden, flaky, buttery croissant slathered with mayo and stacked with tasty ham and thick slices of Swiss cheese, and what appeared to be a leaf layered between cardboard. I frowned, reluctantly choosing the leaf.

Thumping down next to Mike and Andy, I compared trays. Mike had two sandwiches instead of one, and had made no attempt to resist the potato salad. Andy's plate held a roast beef sandwich – the lettuce and tomato carefully removed – an impressive mound of chips, and three giant peanut butter cookies. Sure, Andy was tall, lean, and athletic. He probably burned more calories in a day than I did in a month. But was this fair? "Want me to get you a cookie, Mom?" he asked, noting my mouth watering.

I growled under my breath.

I nibbled a celery stick without even the saving grace of a dab of ranch dressing on the end.

Surprisingly, the sandwich was good. I could actually taste the oaty grains in the wholesome bread, and the crisp freshness of the vegetables. A stem of plump grapes, and I actually felt full. Yeah, I still wanted to leap up and lick the cookie crumbs off Andy's plate, but I resisted. I victoriously lobbed my empty paper plate into the trash. *One small step for dieting-kind.*

On the way home Andy leaned forward in his

seat. "So, did you like the college?" A rare request for parental input.

Mike commented on the attractive campus, modern facilities, competitive athletic program.

"I know!" Andy said. "Maybe I'll make the baseball team."

Wait a minute: it was nice to visit, but really, was he seriously thinking about attending that place ... three hours away from home ... without me? Of course, I knew that this was the expected outcome of the college application process, but it was all getting too close for comfort. This would mean the nest was truly empty. Bad idea. There must be a way to stop this.

"Sure, the college looks great," I said. "And what a comprehensive course catalog." Couldn't hurt to remind him of the academics. "Those classes look intense. You'll have to study night and day to keep up with that."

Mike glanced over and frowned.

Was I dashing Andy's enthusiasm by suggesting a negative? I had nothing against the university, or any other college he'd applied to, but the thought of my youngest so close to leaving home panicked me. By emphasizing the school's demanding academic reputation, perhaps I could suggest the folly of flying the nest.

I scolded myself; that was no way to think. I might not be ready, but Andy was fully prepared to take this step. My job was to make that easier. It wasn't fair to shove my insecurities and worries into his backpack.

"Of course you'll do fine," I added. Damage control.

All at once I craved some vanilla ice cream; the familiar, uncomplicated flavor, the texture so easy and smooth on my tongue, the cool, comforting richness. "Let's swing by the market on the way home!"

By the time we pulled into the parking lot, however, I'd changed my mind. We would not buy ice cream today. I might not be able to stop my children growing up, but I could change the way I dealt with it. I grabbed a cart from the nearby park. Mike joined me, but Andy opted to stay in the car, feet resting against the front seat headrest, iPod earplugs in place.

The first aisle was the produce section. Easy enough. Mike looked amused as I tossed four bagged salads into the cart. "We're going to eat all that?" he asked.

"Yup." I made my way to the bins of vegetables. "The vet said that Kelly should eat carrots," I said, grabbing a two-pound bag of the baby-sized variety.

"Aren't dogs carnivores?"

"Not dogs on diets, and anyway, they're omnivores."

The next aisle proved more difficult. Cereal. "Isn't this what we use?" Mike asked, pulling down my favorite brand. We studied the nutritional label. High in both sugar and fat.

"Put it back," I sighed.

"Granola sounds healthy." But when we checked the label, it contained far too many calories and scads of fat, and that was for just half a cup. "How much do you suppose we pour into a bowl?" Mike asked.

I didn't know, but it surely was more than that tiny measuring device in my kitchen.

Analyzing each product took time. When we finally hit the third aisle Mike resorted to commando guy shopping, stopping at the head of each row to see if we needed anything, rather than proceeding leisurely up and down the lane to carefully examine the goods. "How about a thick, juicy steak?" he asked.

What was it with guys and steak?

"I don't think too much red meat is good for us."

"Frozen french fries?"

"Nothing with the word 'fried'."

"Frozen pizza?"

"No!"

"It's not fried," he justified.

As much as I felt I knew what *not* to buy, I was clueless about what we should purchase. We checked out with lettuce, apples, some healthy-sounding cereal (that looked a bit like

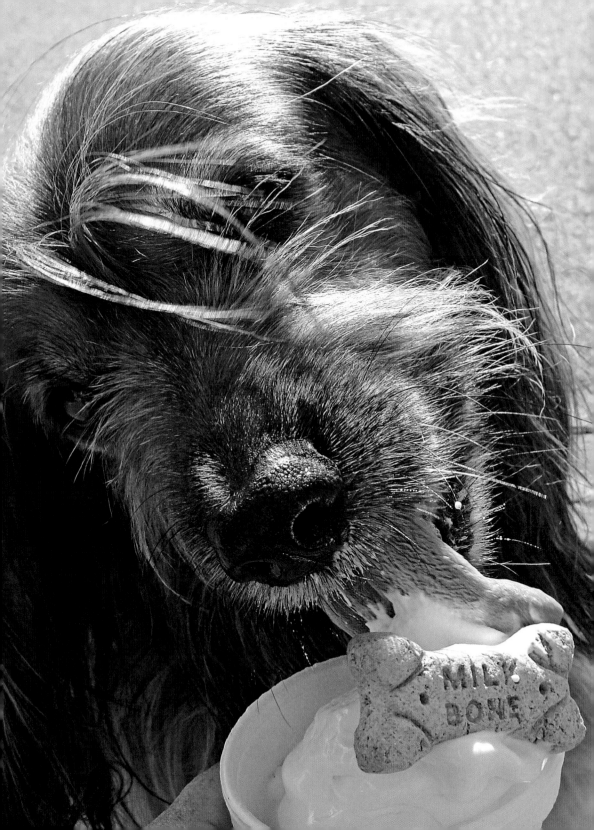

I even introduced Kelly to the joys of ice cream.

rabbit pellets), turkey breast from the deli. And a package of Oreos.

"How'd that get in there?" Mike asked.

I shrugged.

He glared, challenging me to put them back.

"They're, uh … for Andy." I held firm.

I snatched the full grocery bag from the checkout counter and headed toward the door, a corner of the blue and white cookie package poking out of the top. "Baby steps," I muttered under my breath.

The next day I waited in the pantry with a sturdy kitchen trash bag gaping open, its recesses ready to consume our undesirables. "This book says you should get rid of all the bad food in your kitchen," I explained as Mike arrived to help. I emptied a canister of white, starchy pasta into the trash.

"Doesn't the book say anything about starving children somewhere?" Mike surveyed the box of cheesy potato mix I was tossing.

"I'll give away everything I can. One bag will go to the food pantry, and you can take some of the goodies to share with the guys at work. But the opened stuff has to go."

"How about if we eat all this food first, and then start dieting later?"

"Today *is* later. You know what Judy told me last week?" My cousin had been going to nutritional counseling since her heart attack and was feeling stronger. "She said, it's better the food goes to waste than to waist." I motioned around my midsection.

"Aha."

I retrieved an open bag of flour and stuffed it into the trash.

"What was wrong with that?" asked Mike.

"It's white," I said. "Apparently we should avoid white food."

"All white food?"

"I dunno. Maybe. Let's see, white flour, white bread, white sugar, white potatoes …" I read from my new nutritional book.

"Baloney." Mike waved his hand dismissively.

"No, baloney's not white," I said, "but we probably can't eat it anyway."

Given the food usually kept in my house, it was a wonder my kids weren't overweight, but Kate was a trim size six, and Andy was tall, fit and active in sports. Kelly and I were the ones who had blimped out – and, truth be told, Mike had added some weight to his middle over the years, too.

I tossed away open bags of potato chips, crackers, cookies, and a half loaf of soft, white bread. "We're supposed to stick to whole grains. You know, wheat or whatever. Not just any wheat though, it has to be whole wheat. Some breads just put in a part of the wheat and call it 100 per cent wheat bread, but that doesn't mean it's whole grain. It's only made from a part of the grain. It's kind of confusing. And you know enriched white flour? That sounds like something positive – enriched – but apparently it's not ideal. It means they've just taken out the healthy ingredients and added back in some vitamins. Better to have healthy stuff the way it comes naturally. That's what this book says, anyway."

"Huh," Mike said, "well it's worth a try." He joined in, scouring the counter top for other offenders. "I guess this candy from Christmas has to go." Before I could intervene, he chucked it into the bag. "And what about these Oreos?" he added.

"They're for Andy," I grumbled.

Mike glanced at the bathroom scale in the middle of the living room. Kelly walked by, giving it a wide berth.

"Kelly has to be weighed;" I said, crouching to scoop her up, "we need to keep track." Wriggling like an autumn leaf in the wind, Kelly slipped from my grip and scooted off to her

Dieting with my dog

favorite hiding place behind the coffee table. Another one of Kelly's endearing qualities – if you wanted her to do something, it was generally the last thing she was inclined to consider doing.

Mike cornered her against the couch and I lifted her. My arms nearly gave out. She was heavier than I thought. I set her on the scale, but with four paws to maneuver onto one small square, something was always hanging off. When I let go enough to get an accurate reading, she took off again.

"How are we going to do this?" Mike chuckled.

I thought of an old Chinese folk tale I'd read for one of my research projects. The villagers had no scale large enough to weigh an enormous elephant, and all the wise men spent many hours trying to come up with a solution. In the end, the emperor's young son saved the day. He suggested putting the elephant in a large boat on the water, and marking where the hull of the ship met the surface of the water. When that was done, the elephant was unloaded and bricks were added, until the weight of the bricks lowered the boat to the same level. When the bricks were weighed, the young boy explained, they would equal the weight of the elephant.

"Where could we get a boat for Kelly?" I asked.

"What?"

"Never mind. I guess I'll just hold her, and deduct my weight."

I chased her around the room, picked her up and stepped onto the scale. Mike helped read the numbers since I couldn't see past Kelly's huge, furry body in front of me.

"Hurry!" I groaned as she struggled in my arms.

Eventually, the calculations were complete. I jotted down her weight; up another pound since the visit to the vet.

Kelly bolted out of the room to avoid a repeat performance. "Getting on a scale isn't *that* traumatic," I sighed.

"It is for *some* girls, dear," Mike responded.

If Kelly's reaction to being weighed seemed extreme, she was even more averse to her new food plan. I opened the pantry bin and scooped out her meal – a new, high quality weight management dog food. This time I measured it: a half cup. The few little kernels that were her allocation pattered into her bowl. Kelly stared at me, waiting for the rest.

"That's it, girl," I said.

By the time I had put away the scoop, Kelly's bowl was empty again.

While I prepared dinner, she followed me around the kitchen, waiting for something delicious to appear from the magic refrigerator.

"No," I said. She cocked her head, perked her ears and fixed me with her big eyes. *The puppy dog face, not fair!*

I selected some of the new veggies we'd bought at the market. "You can have one of these." I tossed Kelly a baby carrot. She sniffed it and left it where it lay on the floor.

I hadn't previously put much thought into what I cooked for my family; just whatever was easy and tasted good. Now, I tried to give some thought to the nutritional value of each item I would serve. I placed skinless chicken in a baking dish, sprinkled on some seasoning, and slid the dish in the oven. With luck it wouldn't taste awful. I turned to the task of making a salad.

"What's for dinner?" Andy asked. He mainly appeared from his room to eat meals, strew dirty socks, and watch college basketball on television.

"Chicken."

"Can I have pizza?" He looked at me. Another puppy dog face. Saving me from caving in, my cell phone chirped and I flipped it open. Kate's cheerful voice greeted me, telling me all about an exciting project at the web design company

"Maybe if I put just the one paw on the scale, no one will notice ..."

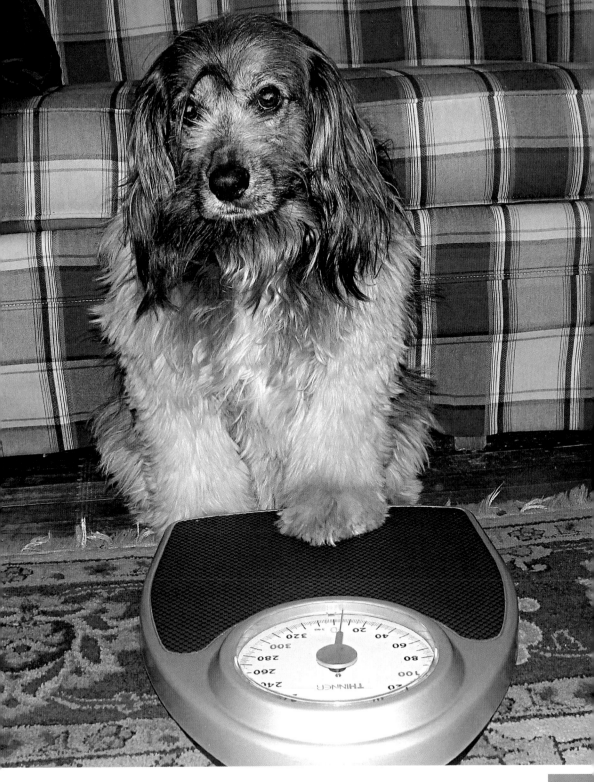

Dieting with my dog

where she worked, and their plans to go to a local theater production. I sat on the kitchen stool, smiling, as she shared her happy life. Out of the corner of my eye I noticed Andy rip open a bag of tortilla chips and disappear to find a game on TV.

"One more thing, Mom," Kate said before we hung up. I could tell by her cautious tone that her announcement wasn't going to make my day. "We're not going to be able to come visit like we'd hoped. Aaron can't get the time off, and I have a million conflicts, and ..."

Kate lived a full day's drive away. With the distance between us, our schedules, Kate's new job, and her husband, Aaron, to take into consideration now, too, the opportunities to see my daughter were limited. Now she was telling me that one of our few planned visits was canceled. I knew the sensitive thing to do was to understand. It wasn't her fault. "I, uh ... ohhh," I stammered.

"We'll definitely do it later, okay? I promise," she said.

I knew that I shouldn't feel upset over something that couldn't be helped (swallow that feeling back down, girl). And why make Kate feel guilty? *Gulp gulp.* I winced, conscious of an actual pain in my stomach. The same pain I had as a girl, when I was the daughter instead of the mother.

Back when I was young, my family had lived in a cramped, one-story house a block from the airport runway. Jets overhead rattled the dishes in the cupboards. Since her divorce, Mom had worked long hours trying to scrape together enough for the bills and take care of me and my two brothers. Sometimes the bills didn't get paid. We didn't have money for the things other kids had, but that didn't matter. I didn't want designer jeans or the latest record album. The only thing I really wanted was food.

School days, my stomach rumbled so that I could barely concentrate until lunch time, when I slid a thick plastic tray along the line, at the end presenting the magic ticket

entitling me to the state's free lunch program. I devoured everything offered by the cafeteria ladies – mystery meatloaf, chopped chicken bits swimming in greasy gravy, lumpy Sloppy Joes.

And, joy of joys, there was even dessert! A small square of brownie or chocolate cake with white icing, maybe, and sometimes even an ice cream sandwich. That was usually on spinach day, each serving a sliver of soggy dark green mush, like from the bottom of a gutter, so thick and slimy that I grimaced as I swallowed. But I ate every bit of that spinach to ensure I wouldn't be denied the ice cream reward that came after.

At home, there would be no snacks in the cupboards. And because Mom worked late, sometimes there was no supper on the table, either. Eventually, and with aching insides, I'd wander into the kitchen and pull down a box of instant mashed potatoes. The little white flakes swelled wonderfully as I stirred in the water.

I spooned the fluffy, white comfort into a bowl and ate it for dinner. Bite by bite, the ache disappeared from my stomach.

What on earth had caused my mind to wander from daughters to mothers to mashed potato? Somehow I knew they were all connected. Love. Relationships. Food.

"We'll get together soon," Kate repeated, and I realized I'd been lost in my thoughts for too long. "Love you."

"Love you," I said, and hung up, keenly aware of that ache.

My first thought of how I'd settle the ache in my stomach was with cookies or pudding. But as I returned to making dinner, washing the produce in the sink, I realized it wasn't hunger that I felt. It was emotion. Disappointment that Kate couldn't come visit. And I couldn't fix disappointment with pudding.

I poised a sharp knife over a stalk of celery and brought it down hard. Chop! I cut right through the thoughts of disappointment. Deprivation: chop. Sadness: chop. Each crispy green splintered into smaller, more manageable sections. I *could* change things. I'd been hungry in the past, but I wasn't hungry any more. I had a supportive family, and, even though Kate was far away, we were still close. Loneliness. Fear of change. Chop chop. I looked into the bowl. By the time I was done, I had a fresh and healthy mixed salad.

Before bed I found an old journal underneath my stack of books on my night table. A tranquil beach scene enhanced the tropical blue cover. I opened the book and studied the blank page before writing.

My past does not define my relationship with food, I wrote. I closed my eyes and put myself on the peaceful blue beach on the book's cover. I let the rhythmic waves wash away everything I thought I knew about food.

Food does not make me:
- *Happy*
- *Comfortable*
- *Safe*

Food does not:
- *Make my life full*
- *Bring Kate home*
- *Keep Andy my baby*
- *Bring me even closer to Mike*
- *Show Kelly love*

Then what is food, I wondered? I felt the tide lap at my toes for a long time before I could complete the thought.

Food is fuel for my body, I wrote. *That's all.*

Agility training

Some of my dieting friends weighed themselves daily, keeping tabs on the numbers before they got out of hand. Others got on the scale only once a week, finding the constant attention to daily fluctuations distracting.

My inclination was to avoid the scale altogether. After about three weeks of shunning fast food and substituting carrots for cookies, however, I tentatively prepared to take a peek.

I'd experimented, and already knew that my scale registered lower on the bare tile floor than the rug. Weigh-ins always took place first thing in the morning before having a bite to eat, and, of course, like any sane woman, I needed to lose every stitch of clothing before checking my weight. My soft, blue nightgown slid into a pool on the floor. Kelly licked my bare toes as I stepped onto the scale. "Cut it out, you're going to throw off the numbers," I said.

I lowered my gaze, my face scrunched up in anticipatory disgust, as if waiting for that scary scene in a movie, the sinister music hinting at what was to come. Looking at the bold red needle on the scale would mean accepting reality. Slowly, the quivering pointer settled on a number. Could it be? I leapt off the scale so fast Kelly scurried out of the room. "Yes!" I cheered, which gave her another scare. "Success!"

For the first time in years, it felt good to be weighed. "Three pounds lost!" I knew they wouldn't show on the outside yet, but already I felt lighter on the inside.

Throwing on some clothes, I skipped down the stairs, Kelly tagging closely behind. Barely out of bed and already the day had taken an upturn! The bottom step, however, proved a challenge. One of Andy's neglected sneakers caught the toe of my fuzzy slipper and my feet flew out from under me. Kelly scooted out of the way as I tumbled onto the wood floor in a heap, my jubilant descent ending in an undiginified landing. No matter how positive things looked one moment, we can always – literally – be brought down to earth.

I eased myself up, rubbing my backside. Kelly's wet nose prodded my ankles helpfully. I nudged the sneakers away with the side of my foot. I could always tell the season by the sports equipment available to trip over at the bottom of the stairs. That day we were transitioning into early spring, the basketball and sneakers mingling with a worn leather baseball mitt and upturned spikes, which were never fun to step on.

Somehow, Andy had developed into an athlete despite my poor example. When he was two, he'd wanted me to play outside with him, so I invented a game I called 'Chair Ball.' My role was to sit in a lawn chair and toss a playground ball, which Andy chased around the yard, with no energy expended on my part. Later, we bought him a pre-school batting tee and a plastic bat. He spent hours hitting a large white Whiffle ball while I sat and watched. Now, he ran, played tennis, lifted weights, shot hoops, and was captain of two sports teams. Mike and I cheered from the stands. I knew there was a correlation between Andy's physical activity and his slim physique. I brushed past his athletic gear. Maybe it was time for me to get in on the game.

Most anyone who has ever tried to lose weight has at some time participated in an exercise class. I'd tried them all. For example, the post-pregnancy Mommy and Baby fitness classes at the community center. Most of us moms were too exhausted to bend and stretch, and the ones who weren't didn't need to attend the class anyway.

Then there was the after-work aerobics group. The limber instructor with a waistline the size of Barbie's led us in agonizing contortions. We echoed her chants as we twisted our bodies into unnatural positions.

"Oh my! Oh my! I've over-developed my thigh!"

"I must, I must, I must firm up my bust."

When Kate was in the tenth grade she invited me to join her cardio-kickboxing classes. I thought it was exciting coiling the red Ace bandage-like wrapping around my wrists and palms. However, for me, that's where the cool factor ended. Lithe young men in flowing cotton pants demonstrated kicks and jabs like angry wind-up toys. Jab, jab, kick, *ugh!* They frightened me because they didn't smile, and their chants were grunts instead of the rhyming encouragement from the after-work fitness lady. Young teens like Kate zipped through the boxing routines with zeal. I wasn't the only older person, but there didn't seem to be another participant who had trouble kicking higher than the dummy's ankles.

During exercises I glanced around the room, hoping to find an equal, perhaps share a secret smile, commiserating in our ineptitude. One grandfather sitting on the side, removing

his clunky leather lace-ups, seemed a likely candidate. Maybe his skill level would even boost my ego. But as he sprang from the metal seat, raised his knee to his chest and thrust a stockinged foot to the top of the punching bag, I knew I was on my own.

I lunged at the dummy with all my might – and pulled a muscle in my inner thigh.

After the thrilling kickboxing classes, I decided to pop a DVD into the player and exercise alone at home instead. On one occasion I worked out with a handsome hunk on the beaches of Hawaii; another I walked in place with a perky instructor, or joined Biggest Loser contestants in jumping jacks. Each time I'd faithfully follow the on-screen routine for a few days, then turn off the TV during the cool down and plop onto the couch with a refreshing drink.

The next time, I'd quit the routine about halfway through.

After that I'd merely look at the DVD cover and set it aside in favor of a non-strenuous sitcom.

Exercising just wasn't for me. I stooped stiffly to pick up Andy's infielder glove from the floor. A stray baseball emerged from underneath. Kelly watched it roll past her feet and yawned. Exercise wasn't her bag, either. Even when the kids tried to awaken some long gone puppy playfulness by chucking one of her toys across the living room, she'd trot just a few feet and then stop to lick a paw: *uh, excuse me, you want me to do what?* I didn't know what spaniels were originally bred for, but, according to Kelly, it wasn't retrieving.

A designer name for her particular mix of Cocker Spaniel, Dachshund and whatever else had yet to be coined, but, observing her behavior, I hovered between 'Napping Spaniel' and 'Long-haired Lazy Hound.'

I retrieved the ball myself and stuffed it into the web of Andy's glove. My past experience

Dieting with my dog

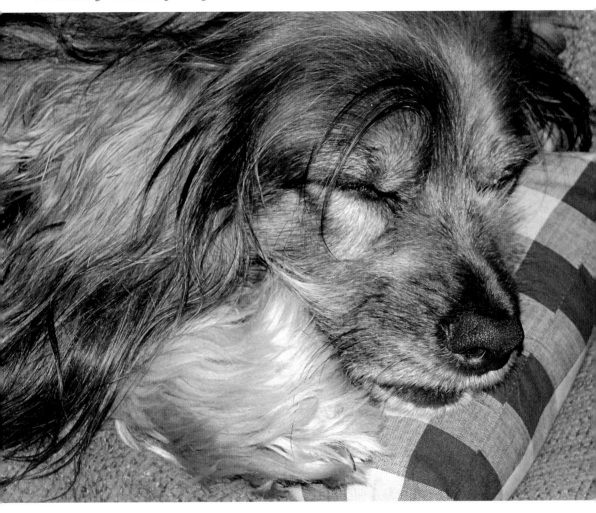

Sweet dreams of sweet treats.

wasn't encouraging, but if I wanted to lose weight, I'd have to try harder.

"I think it's time to get a little exercise," I told Mike that night over the new turkey burgers we'd started eating. They weren't bad at all.

"What about that aerobics class you used to take?"

"Hard on my knees."

Kelly begged under the table. I offered her a baby carrot from my plate. She snatched it from my hand and ran off into the living room.

"She likes them," I observed.

"Umm hmm." Mike took a bite of carrot himself. "Maybe you could look into that new fitness club in town."

"Too expensive."

"Get a treadmill?"

"Where would we put it?"

Mike smiled. "Maybe you don't want to exercise."

Leave it to a guy to see things in black or white. Of course I didn't want to exercise.

However, I'd come to the conclusion that it was what I needed to want. Didn't that make sense?

"Well, there's one exercise I bet you can't dismiss," Mike challenged. "Walking. It's free, easy, and requires no special equipment."

But Mike was wrong. Not only *could* I dismiss walking – I already *had*.

I used to take walks around the neighborhood. In one of my shortlived weight loss sprees I'd laced up my sneakers, hitched Kelly to her leash and hit the pavement. Kelly's tail had waved like a banner flapping in the breeze. Her nose lifted high, taking in the mossy green scent of spring.

We'd strolled to a little park not far from my home, about a mile away by the highway on-ramp that crossed over the river. Kelly wandered at the end of her leash along a steep, sloping bank. Watching her curious exploration, I didn't notice anything else around us until a hulking shape, a dark blur, shot straight toward us. Ears flat, teeth bared … it was a dog – a really big dog.

Ordinarily, I'm not afraid of dogs. But when I saw that huge, vicious-looking beast barreling straight at us, I almost jumped into the river. And considering industry along the riverside had turned the water into a polluted mess, a dip wasn't something to contemplate without substantial provocation.

In the large, grassy expanse where we were there wasn't even a scrawny sapling to shield us. I tightened my grip on Kelly's leash, terrified my cute little pooch was about to serve as an appetizer for the lunging behemoth, with me as the main course. But Kelly forged ahead, her hair standing on end all the way from her neck to the tip of her long, feathery tail. She wasn't afraid at all. She thought she could take that bad boy. "No!" I called, tugging her back.

As the menacing dog bore down, I froze in terror.

Then, a young man in a hoodie sweatshirt appeared at the crest of a hill. A commanding whistle rang out. The burly dog stopped, glared as us over his shoulder, and bolted back to his human.

Kelly and I made it home in record time. I sank into my easy chair and clasped a hand over my racing heart. No way would we venture near that park again. Maybe no place was safe; I'd seen other loose dogs around, in the alleys and behind the railroad tracks. Even on my very own street I'd noticed a big, angry dog dragging a broken length of chain. He could eat us for lunch! My stomach twisted as I recalled stories of mistreated, mishandled fighting dogs. I hefted Kelly onto my lap and held her protectively. "No more walks for us, girl."

Instead, I let Kelly run around in the back yard. Sure, it would be beneficial to get outside and walk again, but recalling the image of the enormous, rampaging dog and its sharp teeth, I only sank deeper into the couch cushions.

Spotting Andy's crumpled batting gloves and stumbling across his sneakers at the bottom of the stairs, however, got me thinking. This emphasized the activity in his life, and the lack of get-up-and-go in my own. And in Kelly's. I looked at her, head propped up on the sofa arm, staring wistfully out the window. Was she missing the walks, the fresh air, the enticing scents? But I didn't dare go outside; one chomp from those dogs and we'd be toast. I turned away guiltily.

The next morning Kelly sat by the front door and looked up at me hopefully. "But Kelly," I tried to explain, "We can't. Those dogs …" Still, as much as I was afraid, maybe … maybe I could do it for Kelly. Somehow, in her deep, brown eyes, I felt her urging me to go outside, for myself as much as for her. *Maybe just a short walk, then.*

I snapped on her leash and looked up and down the street twice before I dared venture past the front steps. "Just one spin around the block," I said as Kelly bounced beside me.

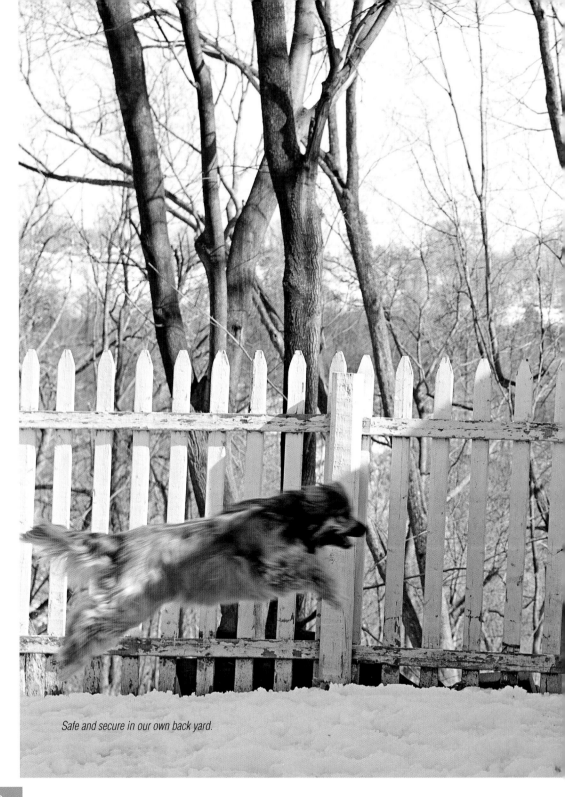

Safe and secure in our own back yard.

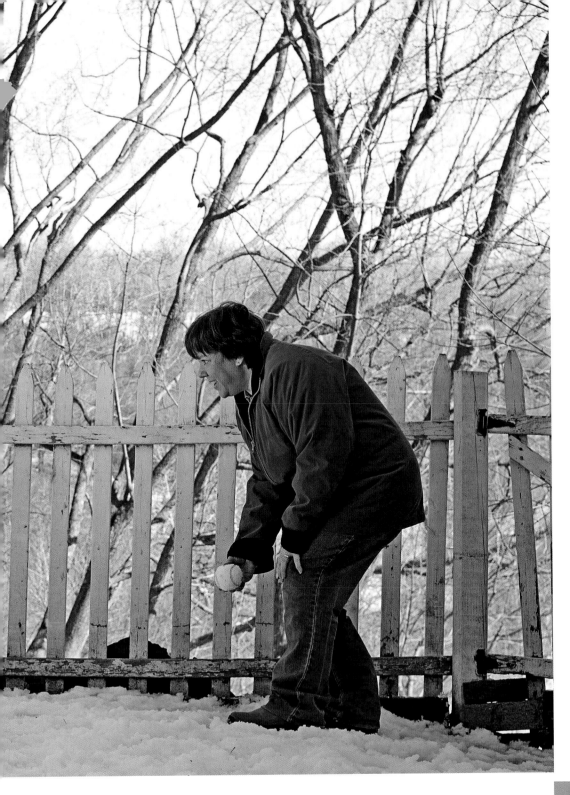

Dieting with my dog

I peered between houses and behind parked cars, ears alert for threatening snarls. *This is no way to walk,* I thought, ready to turn back. Kelly, however, trotted eagerly ahead, pulling me along behind her, unconcerned about what might lie around the corner. She wasn't letting that close call in the park prevent her from enjoying her outing. Actually, when we had encountered that huge dog, she'd faced it bravely, ready to use whatever strength she had to run him off.

Now it was my turn to protect her. I picked up a strong stick lying on the ground. If we did encounter anything dangerous, I could use the stick to try to fend off an attack. Shoulders back, face forward, I strode ahead. This was better. This felt good!

Then, from behind me came the scratching of paws on the pavement. A raspy snort; a menacing warning. Every muscle in my body tensed. Oxygen refused to enter my lungs. I spun around, only to see my fear realized: a loose dog – coming at us.

The terrifying canine stood about ankle high. Long, caramel fur fell around its pushed-in nose and dainty ears, and a pink bow adorned the top of its head. A little rhinestone-studded collar encircled its neck. Four tiny paws scampered at our feet. "Yip!" it said.

My anxiety was released in laughter so explosive I nearly fell over. Kelly casually sniffed the miniature dog. The pup gave one last yip and left, and we continued on our way.

Kelly fell asleep when we returned home, but not the bored napping that usually took up so much of her day. No, this was a deep rest resulting from healthy exertion.

And I felt good, too.

Since Andy got his driver's license, Mike and I no longer spent our evenings waiting for a phone call requesting our convenient pick-up services. If attending a school event, like a concert or play, invariably Andy would become bored and want to come home early. When hanging at a friend's house, however, you never knew when he'd call it a night. Because he didn't attend the local school, none of his friends lived in the neighborhood, but instead, twenty or more miles away. When we'd get the call, "Come get me now," it could take twenty or thirty minutes to get ready and be there. "Why couldn't you call me twenty minutes before you needed to leave?" I'd ask. That never worked.

So, with free time to ourselves that particular night, Mike and I decided to watch a DVD. He slid the disk into the player and sank onto the couch beside me.

The movie was about athletes: runners. I marveled at the characters on the screen, clad in white t-shirts and shorts, sprinting across a smooth sand beach. "How can they enjoy running all the time?" It was enough for me just walking around the block.

"It's their passion," Mike said. He'd seen *Chariots of Fire* many times.

"I know. But runners always look in pain and exhausted. Doesn't look like fun to me."

I was still doubting the thrill of all that running when the camera pulled in tight on one of the main characters, his face soft yet intense as he spoke. "I believe that God made me for a purpose," he said, "but He also made me fast, and when I run, I feel His pleasure." Those beautiful words swirled in my head as the music swelled. If God made me for a purpose, I thought, it surely wasn't for running. On the other hand, what if I did get up and move? What if I actually pushed my body in order to get fit? Would I then feel His pleasure?

I wanted to. At that moment I knew I wanted to.

The next morning Kelly was in her favorite spot again, sprawled across the back of the couch, chin resting on her paws, listless and bored. What kind of life was this for a dog? For me, too. One walk didn't mean anything. We had to do that every day.

"Come on," I called, "Time to get moving."

Kelly moved slowly off the couch, stopping to stretch halfway. I put a little more pep in my voice. "Hop to it, you couch potato. Let's go!"

Her ears perked as I reached for the leash. When I opened the front door and the fresh air hit us, her nose lifted. Her head swung back and forth as she scanned the street. Then she nearly pulled me down the front steps as she lunged for the sidewalk.

This time no dog, not even a Pomeranian, crossed our path. We walked farther than I thought we would – or could. Noticing how much Kelly enjoyed herself, it wasn't as hard to motivate myself to keep going.

The next day rain pelted against the side of the house and gusts of wind rattled the old window panes. Mike swished a dish rag in the sink while I peeked out the back door. Forget it. I'd rather help Mike wash the dishes, a chore I generally avoided like a tofu sandwich. "We're not walking today."

"Can't you think of something else to do?" Mike asked. "Like jumping jacks?"

"Suppose so. But what about Kelly?"

Hearing her name, she wandered into the kitchen and sat in front of the refrigerator. I spotted a tennis ball and bounced it on the floor. She yawned.

"You've got to *sell* it," said Mike. He took the ball, waved it in front of Kelly's face, then quickly pulled it away. He admired the toy as if it were a great treasure, raising his voice in mock excitement. "Look at this! Isn't it great? Do you want it? You want it, girl?"

This caught Kelly's attention. Though not quite ready to buy, she was definitely in the market. Mike released the ball and it flew across the kitchen. He only had to pounce a few exaggerated steps forward for Kelly to charge, full tilt, after the missile. Tail wagging, she misjudged her braking ability and skidded into the far wall, yet ended up with the prize; a fuzzy tennis ball that had collected lint, hair and dirt along its journey. All the better, as far as a dog's concerned.

Joining in the game, I tossed the ball into the living room. Kelly chased, losing it between a basket of magazines and the loveseat. I knelt to retrieve it. "What's this?" I asked, my hand falling upon something cold and hard. I pulled out a shriveled baby carrot. "Kelly!" Behind the basket were even more carrots. Apparently, she wasn't convinced about her new snack.

I tossed away the shriveled veggies. Some day maybe she'd appreciate healthy food, just as she'd come to enjoy physical activity. After our rousing game of fetch, I picked up the morning paper, folded over to the classifieds.

"Look. A used elliptical machine for sale." I showed Mike the ad. "It says it's compact. We can fit it right into the corner of the living room. It's in good condition. A really good price. What do you say? We could go pick it up tomorrow after Andy's baseball game."

I wasn't expecting quick agreement. Surely, Mike remembered as well as I did the graveyard of unused fitness equipment in the basement. The old exercise bike, clunky and out of date, that was used for about a week; where's the fun in pedaling without getting anywhere? The bulky plastic steppers, a series of rubber-treaded platforms that stacked to new heights with each level. But that form of torture wasn't any more appealing than walking in place. Nearby languished a pile of old exercise VHS tapes. *Sweating to the Oldies. Feel the Burn. Buns of Steel.* And yes, *VHS,* even though that technology was long since out of date.

Mike looked at me, all mussed up and sweaty from playing with the dog, and grinned. "Sure," he said.

The next day we got ready to go to the baseball game. Andy had met up with the team earlier. I stood ready to go, Kelly by my side.

"Uh, what are you doing?" Mike asked.

"Wouldn't it be nice to take her to the game?"

Dieting with my dog

"Not really," he answered. We'd tried taking Kelly places before. She shed hair all over the car seats, panted smudges on the windows, and tugged at the leash, demanding constant attention.

"She needs to get more exercise. It'll be fun."

Mike sighed as I deposited Kelly on the back seat of the van and slid the door closed. She squeezed between the armrests and climbed into my lap in the front seat, as usual. Mike turned the key, defeated.

"I'm going to pay attention to the game," he said. "Don't let her distract anyone."

"She won't."

We sat in folding lawn chairs to the left of the backstop. About halfway through the first inning, my hands had hardened into arthritic fists from clenching the leash. I pushed Kelly into a down position, hoping she'd settle in and lie contentedly in the grass by our feet. Instead, she pulled toward the field, now apparently overly-interested in balls. I shuddered to imagine the pitcher going into his windup, his concentration intense, only to be startled by a sudden shrill bark as he released the ball.

"Shhhh," Mike warned.

Kelly fussed like a spoiled toddler, attempting to wedge her flailing limbs onto my lap. I wrangled her to the ground beneath my chair.

"Andy's up," said Mike, trying to concentrate on the game.

Andy stepped out of the on-deck circle and approached the plate. Kelly's ears perked and she tugged harder. Her whining grew in intensity.

"Interference," Mike whispered in my direction, pretending to be the ump. He frowned at Kelly. "If you don't behave, you're ejected."

The first pitch: low and outside. Andy stepped back and took a practice swing. The next pitch was a change-up. The bat cracked. Kelly barked.

The sight of the ball whizzing across the field was too much for her, and she bolted from under my chair. The leash in my hand tightened. In a flash of horror, I watched the leash tangle around the legs of the chair. Kelly took off. The chair collapsed. I somersaulted onto the grass. Mike pretended he didn't know us. I jumped up and raced after Kelly, stumbling and panting. Finally, I caught hold of the trailing leash and reclaimed my charge, hiding my face from the other spectators. We skulked back to the car to wait out the rest of the game.

Fortunately, Andy was safe on first.

After that, we figured Kelly and baseball were best kept separate. Walking in the neighborhood would have to do for her. Still, some days I just wanted to sit on the couch instead of going out. Why was it so difficult to motivate myself to do something I knew was good for me?

The elliptical machine, for example, was supposed to be beneficial. Squeezed into the corner of the living room beside the loveseat, the machine whooshed enthusiastically some days and sat neglected others. The first time I got up on the equipment, I pushed the long, wide treads in a smooth pedaling motion. It felt effortless – for precisely three minutes, that is. After that, it felt more like wading through quicksand in cement boots (even though the resistance was on the lowest setting).

The contraption was positioned in such a way that it was possible to watch the television, in order to distract ourselves with an interesting program. The larger distraction for me, however, was the couch. I noticed it out of the corner of my eye while pedaling, and every fiber in my body wanted to jump off the annoying machine and snuggle into the soft, comforting cushions I knew and loved.

For the first week, I could manage a maximum of eight minutes on the machine. I pumped my legs, pushed my arms back and forth, and with each step felt my muscles turn to jelly. In fact, they weren't even muscles, they were the opposite of muscles, whatever that

Kelly supervises my workouts.

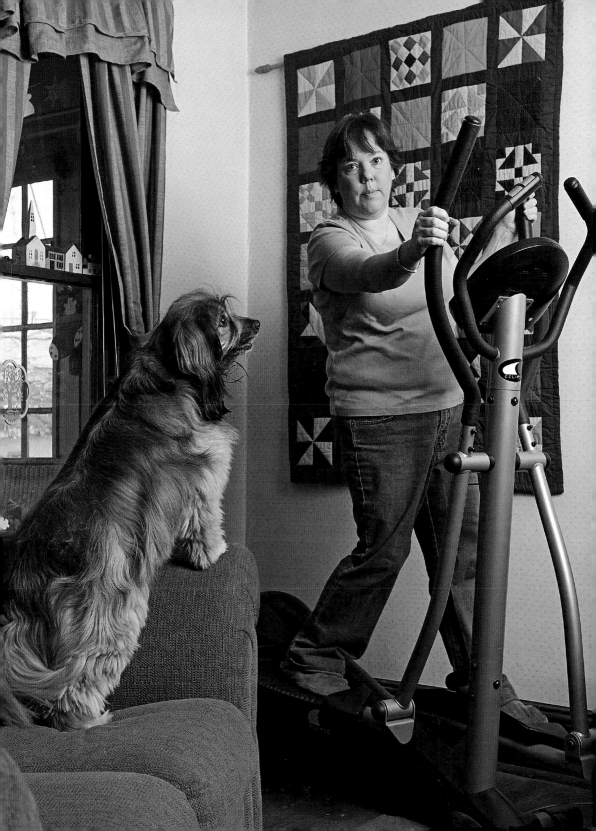

Dieting with my dog

was. Tissue? Spaghetti? I looked longingly at the sofa, its voluptuous cushions beckoning to me. Elliptical machines were not soft and cozy. Why had no one thought to equip the blasted device with a padded seat and pillow?

Eight minutes was a start, but my goal was to work out for at least 20 minutes every day. To be honest, I was searching for the minimum amount of time I'd have to spend in order to achieve at least moderate calorie burn, and eight minutes didn't quite cut it. I looked it up; eight minutes working out, at my pace, could burn off one Sun Chip. Unfortunately, I planned to eat more than one bite-sized, low fat multigrain crunchy snack per day. So the eight-minute mark was the make or break point. If I could survive past that, I knew I had a chance.

Each day I tried to add one more minute to my time. How could 60 seconds tick away so achingly slowly? Maybe I needed to stop watching the time readouts. I flicked on the television, hoping it would be the distraction I needed.

"You're doing pretty well with that thing," Mike said one night. "I think I'll give it a try." He climbed on and pumped the treads. Faster than I had, too.

Maybe accountability would help. I got out a notebook. "Let's keep track of how long we go." I set the pad and a pen on the end table. Mike's participation had a positive effect on me. Every day when I saw his entry, I wanted to do more. If he could do 15 minutes, so could I. I just had to get over that frustrating eight-minute roadblock.

"Who would have guessed you were so competitive?" Mike asked, wiping the sweat from his brow.

"I'm not," I said, taking my turn as he climbed off. "Now, how far did you say you just went?"

The elliptical resided in plain view from my desk in the corner; an unavoidable reminder. During the work week, when it was time for a break, I started a new routine. Dr Phil was on

TV at 3pm. I put away my work, switched on the television, and climbed onto the elliptical.

"What are you doing?" Mike asked one afternoon when he called around that time.

"Phillipticalling," I replied.

The show was engaging enough to take my mind off counting down the minutes. Hopefully, I'd make it to at least eight minutes without giving up.

When I looked at the display on the handlebars, it read 17. Not bad! My pace quickened; I could do more, too!

Later, Mike dug out some old hand weights and pumped them back and forth to add to his workout. I made extra trips up and down the stairs. We parked farther away from the mall entrance – on purpose. This was all starting to make sense. A few toning exercises were fitted into my routine, as well as more playtime with Kelly. And, whenever we could, Kelly and I went out and strolled around the block. We both wanted to.

Saturday night and Andy was out again. I couldn't quite get used to not being involved in his plans, taking a back seat instead of being taxi driver to his schedule. I wasn't totally out of the picture, though, as he still called to let me know where he was and when he'd return. I still waited up for him to pull into the driveway safe and sound. But times when he was away, and Mike and I were home with no kids in the house, made me restless. I was too aware that it was practice for the real thing, the real empty nest, that we'd have in a few short months.

And the quietness was unsettling, too. No clomping on the stairs. No pop music I was too old to understand thumping from behind the bedroom door. No rundown of the latest sports contest on TV.

Until recently, our social calendar had revolved around the kids' activities. Not just driving them around, but also attending school assemblies and parent meetings, volunteering on school committees, not to mention supporting Andy's basketball and baseball teams. That meant two or three games a week, plus tournaments. When he added community league baseball to his schedule, multiple games consumed most Saturdays, too. Occasionally, Mike and I got together with friends, went to a movie or a church activity, but for the most part the kids were our social lives and there wasn't time – or energy – for anything more.

Even nights when Andy was out, Mike and I often spent our together-time talking about schedules and kids. Lately, college plans consumed our free moments. Where would he decide to attend? Could we afford it? What supplies would he need? What was the best meal plan? That night, however, we were momentarily talked-out about college so Mike scanned the shelves for a DVD to watch. "What sounds good to you?"

Watching movies at home, with Kelly curled up beside us on the couch, was usually as much excitement as we could handle in a night. But, as I watched Kelly yawning listlessly on the rug, I thought this was not the best we could do. She was like a mirror, reflecting the tedium of inactivity that had permeated our nights. "You know what?" I said, surprising even myself. "I don't really feel like watching a movie tonight. I feel like taking a walk instead. It's a nice night. Wanna come?" I could barely think of a time in all our years together we'd gone out for a walk instead of staying in. It hadn't even crossed my mind before.

Mike scratched his neck. "Guess so." He pushed the DVD he'd selected back onto the shelf.

We strolled down the street side by side. I held Kelly's leash and she trotted along eagerly, no pulling or straining. The warm evening air was damp and fragrant with the blossoming of early spring. Two cats yowled amiably as they snuck between the hedges.

We looked up at the moon and Mike squeezed my hand.

Old dog, new tricks

It was my birthday and I wanted cake. I'd had the elaborate concoction planned for nearly a year; even ripped a picture from the pages of a magazine. Four layers of chocolate cake with white buttercream frosting spread thickly over the top and sides; the towering work of art covered completely in colorful dots of blue, green, red and yellow M&M's. My mouth watered just thinking about it.

My new diet, however, meant I'd never see this masterpiece outside of my dreams. What was a birthday without cake?

When my kids were growing up, the perfect birthday cake took weeks of planning. No store-bought, pre-decorated jobs for me. This was not about baking; I rushed through the tedious cake mix instructions on the back of the box. The thrill was in crafting and building. Although I couldn't match the smoothness of the frosting, or the perfect symmetry of a bakery's piped-on letters, the reward of decorating a unique dessert for each child was mine alone.

Some of my creations turned out brilliantly. Like Andy's treasure chest cake: a chocolate-frosted base with a slab of cake propped up to resemble the lid of an open trunk, diamond-shaped ring pops and gold foil-covered coins spilling out from within. Andy could hardly bear to ruin it by cutting a slice. "Wow, Mom, cool!"

Other attempts were less successful. Kate's 'bunnies in a garden' cake was crafted with an over-zealous amount of confectionary sugar frosting, dyed what turned out to be garish Incredible Hulk green. Pink flowers morphed into puddles. Little plastic rabbits tipped over or disappeared completely into the mountains of frosting. Bunny garden party meets *The Blob*. Still, every birthday I attempted a new confection to mark the special occasion.

I'd even been known to make birthday cakes for my dogs. When I was little, I made mud cakes out in the back yard for my hound dog, Happy. Sometimes, I also drew him a card. He'd sit beside me watching my every move, as if he actually wanted these offerings. Since he'd been abused and abandoned, he was probably grateful for any act of love, I guess.

Although I'd outgrown mud cakes (which would never do for Kelly anyway), I still marked her special day. Her birthday cakes consisted of home-created recipes, special dog-appealing concoctions that still looked like mud but apparently tasted like prime rib, bone-shaped biscuits decorating the top.

"Should we throw her a party?" I'd asked Andy when Kelly first joined our family. "Invite some dog friends?"

Silly, maybe, but to me a birthday meant a celebration. Little kids needed games and party favors, but after the last tail was pinned on the donkey and the balloons had popped, they expected a sugar hit in the form of rich, gooey cake. As we get older, of course, there are no games and often no parties, and all that's left to mark the day is a dessert with glowing candles. I always preferred one candle for each year, not those cheating number-shaped candles. Even when the blazing candles represented a possible fire hazard. I liked to see my name written out, too, *Happy Birthday, Peggy,* to emphasize the significance of the day. And when that cake was carried out on a pretty platter with everyone singing, off-key or otherwise, I would beam broadly. This was my day, it said so in frosting, and I was special.

"I didn't get you a cake," Mike confessed as we came in from walking Kelly, the afternoon of my 47th birthday.

"That's okay," I said.

"You told me not to."

"I know."

He paused, smiling gently. "Go on and get ready. We'll go out to dinner. Anywhere you want."

I wasn't one to focus on age. I love birthdays so much, age isn't usually a factor. This birthday, however, I couldn't help feeling old. My hair was graying. Andy had even pointed out a few frightening chin hairs. I wore bifocals for reading and computer work. My kids were right. I was old. How old were *my* parents when I went away to college? Practically dinosaurs.

"I don't know if I should still give you this," Mike said before we went out to the restaurant. He handed me a small wrapped box.

"You already gave me gifts!" Earlier that morning he and Andy had presented me with the brand new novel I'd been pining for, a pot of daisies, and a beautiful necklace. "What could it be?"

I removed the pretty silver bow, ripped open the paper, and pulled out a cellophane bag. Inside were special, custom-printed M&M's, in my favorite color; green. Each one was personalized. I held them close to examine the writing. 'I love Peg,' they all read.

"I ordered them before you were really dieting …"

"Oh, Mike," I gushed, reaching over to give him a hug. "They're perfect." I clutched the candy, smiling. Some food could make you feel good without taking a single bite.

That night we entered the darkened dining room of a nice restaurant, one we reserved for special occasions. On a shoestring budget, we mostly hit fast food chains in the past. When the kids were little, we could order entire meals for less than two dollars each. In their teens, we did pretty well off the dollar menu. Cheap, and all stuff we knew they'd eat. I loved fast food, too. I'd have a double burger with toasted bun, strips of sizzling bacon, slices of cheese and mayonnaise. We'd each have our own fries. No sharing. Whenever I saw the four bulging cardboard envelopes of hot french fries spilling out onto the plastic tray, the enormity of the quantity hit home. A wet pool of grease bloomed across the paper tray liner. Still, those crispy golden fries *were* delicious ...

At the restaurant, there were no paper wrappers or cardboard containers. The three of us even stepped it up for the occasion: I had on a new, emerald green top and Mike wore a sports coat. Even Andy ditched his major league tee in favor of a nice, clean dress shirt.

We sat at a corner booth, soft candlelight dancing from a glass lantern in the center. Deep reds and rich cherry walls gave the room a refined feel.

The waiter handed us large, folded menus. I tried to open mine without knocking over my wine glass, or disrupting the extra pieces of silverware crowding my place setting. This was my first time eating out since I began my diet. I'd had some significant weight loss by now, and I wanted to continue making the right choices.

Dieting with my dog

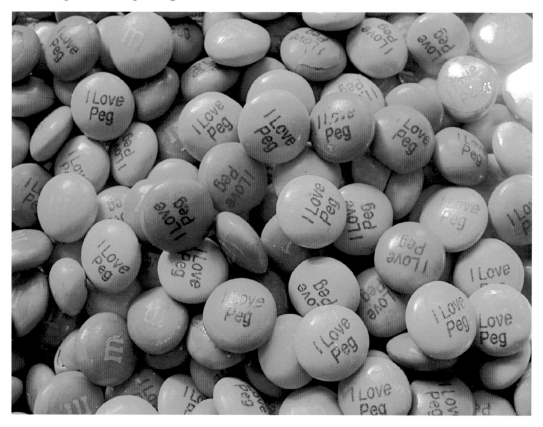

These candies actually turn out to be good for me!

But it was my birthday! Couldn't I also enjoy myself?

I read the entrées carefully, struggling between caution and indulgence.

Ordinarily, my selections would have been easy. Creamy fettuccini Alfredo, dripping with cheese sauce and garlic. Warm, crusty bread spread thick with butter. Dessert, without a doubt. Molten lava cake oozing with hot fudge, cool, rich, vanilla bean ice cream on the side.

All diet disasters!

In the end, I chose a salad, dressing on the side, grilled chicken instead of the fried, seasonal vegetables, and no dessert. Although presented artfully, the food looked sad on my plate. The chicken was good, but as I lifted a healthy forkful to my mouth the waiter walked past with my meal of choice, destined for some other lucky diner.

We picked a date at random, our best guess, to celebrate Kelly's birthday. When we adopted her from the rescue shelter, we were told she was about a year old, but I pegged her as a little younger, about 9 months old, based on her behavior and how much growing she did.

For her earliest birthdays, we'd showered her with extra treats and cookies, and of course that cake made of rice and cheese and whatever yummy leftovers I thought she'd enjoy. This year, I wanted to do something better. I still liked the idea of a party, but logistically, an assembly of dogs gathered in our small house didn't seem practical.

The morning of the big day, Kelly jumped onto the bed and burrowed under the covers like every other morning. "I'm taking a break from work today, Kelly," I said. "This day's going to be just for you. We'll spend it however you want."

We skipped downstairs and I opened the back door. She ran outside and sniffed around in the fresh spring air for longer than usual as I didn't call her back inside when it suited me. Later, when she dropped a tennis ball at my feet, I tossed it to her repeatedly, until she was ready to lie down and call it quits. Instead of typing at the computer, I stretched out on my chair with a book, Kelly by my side.

When Mike and Andy arrived home, we all sang *Happy Birthday* and gave Kelly a present: a plastic jug that dispensed treats, but only after she flung it around and expended plenty of energy playing. Finally, it was time for the 'cake' – a lump of tender, cooked chicken breast scraps, mixed with premium carob-chip canine cookies. Six tiny baby carrots stuck up on top like candles. Six years old: my big girl.

Another special birthday that year was Judy's. She'd recovered from her heart attack, faithfully attended rehab with nutritionists and exercise classes, and was doing better than ever with her weight loss. "I actually feel better than before," she'd told me earlier on the computer. "I can do more. I have more energy. With the blockage in my artery cleared, it's like I'm a new me."

We drove the two-hour journey to the busy steakhouse for her party. Judy stood among her friends and family, cheeks glowing from all the attention. She'd lost a considerable amount of weight, and although she still had some to go, looked like the new woman she'd described.

"Peggy!" she cried when she spotted me, running up to give me a big hug. "Look at you, you've lost so much!" We talked at least weekly and I'd been reporting on my progress, but we hadn't actually seen each other in months.

"Happy Birthday! So glad you're feeling better. You look fantastic." I didn't want to keep her from her other guests, but now, seeing her concrete dieting results, I wanted to find out more about her strategies face-to-face. "How do you keep it off?" I asked, after managing to corner her for a few minutes.

"Basically, I eat the same thing every day. I don't trust myself to make choices any more."

The same meals every day didn't sound very appealing to me, but everyone is different. Although it wasn't a strategy I wanted to try, I was curious. "What do you have for breakfast?" I asked.

"The same brand of high fiber cold cereal every day. And lunch is always fat-free light yogurt, a turkey sandwich with fat-free cheese and two pickle slices." She described the veggie-packed chef's salad she made for dinner and snacks of fruit and sugar-free pudding. "That's it. If I don't have to think about options, I don't have to worry about temptation."

For Judy, this worked. She didn't deviate from low-fat, low-calorie options; not even a swipe of mayo on her sandwich. And I knew she was exercising every day, too. For her efforts, she was rewarded with a slow and steady pound-a-week weight loss.

"But what about holidays? Birthdays? How do you handle those?"

"Poorly," she answered quietly, and I knew she felt the challenge of special occasions just like me. No doubt, parties would always be difficult.

Mike and I stocked up at the spotless salad bar, brimming with crisp peppers, sliced mushrooms, broccoli, even chilled beets and sweet peas. Many of these salad options were new to me, since I'd mainly only tried uninspired iceberg lettuce topped by a slice of tomato. By contrast, this salad – a little low-fat balsamic vinaigrette drizzled over the top – brimmed with new tastes and textures just begging to be experienced – delicious. We each ordered a small steak, and saved half to take home for

Dieting with my dog

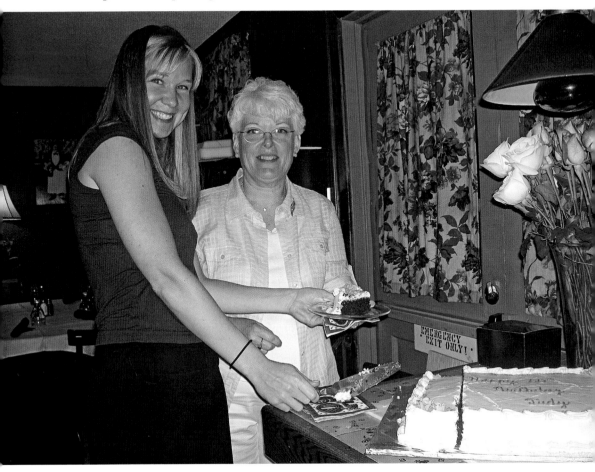

Judy, with daughter Sarah, and the main event.

later. I was so busy catching up with friends and relatives, I didn't think about being hungry.

Then the big moment arrived: the birthday cake – fancy, marbled sponge with white icing and lavish lavender lettering – appeared amid singing and clapping. Judy cut the first slice. I thought of my own birthday without a cake, and whimpered at the thought of missing out on this one, too. Was deprivation the key?

In the past, even the thought of a celebratory dessert made me feel as if wrapped in a sweet embrace, and eating as much as I could meant getting more of that love. Turning it down for the sake of dieting left me feeling like the kid at school with an empty shoebox on Valentine's Day. Where was that love? Maybe a little taste would do the job; I asked for just a sliver.

In the past, a slice would have been wolfed down in several quick bites. Followed by a second piece. This time, however, I slowly slid a dainty forkful of cake into my mouth.

The icing touched my tongue and the inside of my cheeks, and I tasted it with every part of my mouth until it melted away and disappeared.

"There's so much left over. Here, take a slice home." The server offered me another plateful.

"No, thanks," I replied. "That was just enough." And it was.

Spring was my favorite time of year, except for one thing. Shedding the heavy layers of winter clothes. Who wanted to show the bulk that lurked underneath? The snow melted, the trees budded, but I still wanted to hide beneath a heavy parka, taking refuge under the camouflaging abilities of a bulky, down-filled coat.

When the weather turned warm and inviting at Easter, though, I was finally ready to wear some pretty spring clothes. I loved Easter Sunday; little girls at church in wide pink bonnets, carrying white plastic purses. Little boys in short pants and plaid bow ties. Easter egg hunts. Bunnies. Rainbow-colored dyed eggs. The sweet smell of spring, the message of hope. And, of course, there's the Easter candy. Baskets of bright jelly beans my kids used to sort by color and count the members of each pile. Miniature chocolates wrapped in pastel foils, candies in the shape of eggs and chicks. Chocolate bunnies with long ears, just asking to be bitten off first. How would I resist them?

Easter morning, I slid into my standard floral holiday dress. Maybe the old-fashioned lace collar aged me a bit, but the dress skimmed over the bulges and flowed to the ankles to keep everything under cover. Actually, it was too loose. I glanced at my silhouette in the mirror; yep, my stomach *was* a little less rotund.

Downstairs, Kelly dashed outside to play in the brisk, fresh air. The grass was still winter-yellow and flat, but here and there little sprigs of new growth popped up and strained toward the sun, and crocus leaves had begun to unfurl as a welcome to the warmth.

For breakfast, I cracked some eggs, separated the yolks and tossed these away. My mom always disapproved of wasting food. She had a point, but why save the yolks for cakes or custards I shouldn't eat? I remembered Judy's mantra: "The food can go to waste, or go to waist." No sense in using up my calories on something as boring as eggs. Whites contained few calories, and no fat or cholesterol, so I could eat the whites of about five eggs compared to one whole egg. Much more filling.

Andy arrived at the breakfast table first. Even though the kids were grown, we still carried out the tradition of filling Easter baskets. Everyone got a different color decorative grass in their basket. Unlike Halloween with its depressing black and gaudy orange, or Valentine's Day with the reds and pinks I never thought went well together, Easter was alive with joyous pastels. Mike received the traditional green grass in his basket. Andy, a boyish light blue. And for me, a soft lavender. Earlier, I'd mailed Kate and Aaron a basket lined with duckling yellow grass.

"Sweet," Andy said, unearthing a large, long-eared chocolate bunny from the center of his basket. With a sleepy smile, he shuffled through the jellybeans, little packages of baseball cards, and peanut butter eggs.

Even Kelly had a little basket. Inside was a new toy and some special low-fat dog treats made with blueberries and pumpkin. New tastes for her to try, too.

Mike arrived, buttoning the top of his dress shirt. He grinned when he saw the table. I was always in charge of filling the baskets and took the task seriously, sprinkling them with our favorite candies and cute traditional sweets. For Mike and me, however, this year I'd had a new idea.

Just behind the arched handles, instead of chocolate bunnies, sat a fat, golden pineapple. The green spiky tops stuck up almost like long ears. Surrounding the pineapple were shiny red apples, bright oranges, plump purple grapes. I beamed at my Easter fruit baskets.

"Good job!" said Mike. He plucked a grape and popped it into his mouth.

Maybe I was getting the hang of holidays.

Treats and retreats

I threw a t-shirt and jeans into the duffle bag, then added a fleece. Although the start of the summer vacation season, Memorial Day weekend could still blow in with a brisk chill. Especially up in the mountains.

"Are you going to pack your swimsuit?" asked Mike. We liked to swim in the lake, but this time of year the weather was iffy.

"Uh … nuh-oh." My tone was snippy.

The water could be frigid, true, but that wasn't the only reason I wouldn't be swimming this time: I wasn't anxious to expose my spare tire and flabby thighs. Sure, I'd lost a dozen or so pounds, but that was a drop in the ocean. And lately, I hadn't been losing anything at all; my weight simply refused to budge. In the mornings, Kelly followed me into the bathroom and eyed the scale as I gingerly stepped on. I shifted my body, hoping it might make a difference to the reading. But the numbers hadn't changed in weeks; I'd reached The Dreaded Plateau.

Every dieter knows about this. Whenever you stop losing weight, people attempt to make you feel better by saying you're probably 'just on a plateau.' While better than gaining weight, The Plateau was frustrating because I still watched what I ate, worked out on the elliptical, and denied myself nightly soft-serve ice cream cones, but without reaping the rewards! The Plateau had chewed away enough at my confidence already. I wasn't about to compound that by modeling a swimming suit.

You'd think guys would understand about gals and swimming suits. Those tiny Lycra garments had to support a boatload of emotional baggage. Every year I'd squeezed into the same modest suit – the suit that said, "Don't look at me, I'm fat." – with the magic tummy panels, low leg line and high back that left everything to the imagination – only nobody wanted to imagine it. I buried my swimsuit in the corner of my dresser. I hated that thing.

At the mall just last week I'd seen a beautiful, rainbow selection of bright yellow bikinis, dazzling raspberry halters, Mediterranean aqua tanks, but, for larger gals, the color of choice is always black. Supposedly, it's 'slimming.' What a lie! There was no slimming a lumpy sausage stuffed into a tight nylon skin. I hated black swimsuits. My swimsuit was black, and I wasn't going to wear it.

Every summer we vacationed at our getaway, a small cabin on a lake up in New York's Adirondack mountains. The cabin – thankfully, with indoor plumbing – had been in my husband's family since he was a young boy. For long weekends and holidays, this was our destination.

Memorial Day weekend was always our first chance to get up there, and I couldn't wait. The peace and quiet, beautiful scenery. Plenty of time to relax; no computer, television, telephones. No distractions.

I grabbed deodorant and an extra toothbrush off my dresser. You didn't need much at the lake. It didn't matter if you put on clothes with holes or forgot to run a brush through your hair. It was camp.

The kids adored vacations at Nan and Pop's place, especially when they were younger. Swimming, boating, undivided attention from their grandparents. The older they got, though, the more difficult visiting became. Kate hadn't had time to pop in since she'd graduated from college. And although he still loved spending time with his grandparents, Andy sometimes took issue with the amenities. The bottom of the lake was mucky, and besides, with his sister away, swimming alone wasn't as much fun. The 20-foot pontoon wasn't exactly a muscle boat. And inside – no television. What if he missed a record-breaking Yankees homerun? Not to mention the absence of internet, and even cell reception out in the boondocks.

Surprisingly, this weekend he didn't complain or suggest staying home. Maybe because it was the last summer before going off to college and he took pity on me, or maybe he really wanted to be with us. A mom can dream.

We stepped out of the van into the fresh mountain air. Smoke curled lazily from the cabin's chimney, and I pictured a snug fire in the old black woodstove inside. Nan and Pop waved from the porch, Nan wrapped in a knobbly-knit cardigan sweater, Pop in his plaid wool shirt. Kelly was the first to greet them, darting out of the van, nearly tugging the leash from my grip. I wished she could have run loose, but her insistence on ignoring the basic recall command made that idea out of the question. Plenty of potential hazards lurked, even out in the country. Although lightly traveled, the road behind the cabin was a two-lane highway. Kelly

had no street savvy, so we didn't dare let her free near a road. Dense marshland beyond the cabin was deep enough to practically consume a small Spaniel; I knew because, more than once, I'd sunk up to my knees in that muck. Tall grasses along the shoreline rustled with whispers of wildlife. And the lake itself tempted with sparkling water and rippling waves. As alluring as everything was, when our dog was outside she had to stay on a long leash for her own safety.

"You look great," Nan said, giving me a hug around my smaller middle. It still felt strange to hear this observation. While this endorsement was encouraging, it also added pressure. Now that my weight loss was noticeable, what would everyone think of me if it stopped? Or if I gained again? My personal struggle was becoming very public.

Kelly bounded around the yard, her tail winding in circles like a helicopter rotor. Ears alert, nose to the ground, she raced from shrub to tree trunk. She stuck her nose in a chipmunk hole, coming back up with a comical snort, clearing rooty soil from her nostrils. This was how it should be for a dog. Excited, engaged in her environment, busy, not lounging around on the back of a couch. Although the smells of the city weren't as intoxicating as those at camp, the mental stimulation Kelly now received from our walks back home was just as important as the physical exercise.

We traipsed into the cabin, greeted by sweet, piney wood smoke. If I'd made the trip blindfolded I would have known exactly where I stood, just from that aroma. When Mike and I were dating he'd taken me to the cabin, and we'd sat up late into the night, talking quietly so we wouldn't wake his parents, stoking the flames in that wood stove, adding birch logs that crackled when they caught fire. The next day we held hands, sitting side by side on the dock in the blazing midday sun. If I closed my eyes it was almost as if time had stood still.

That night we lounged around the slim-

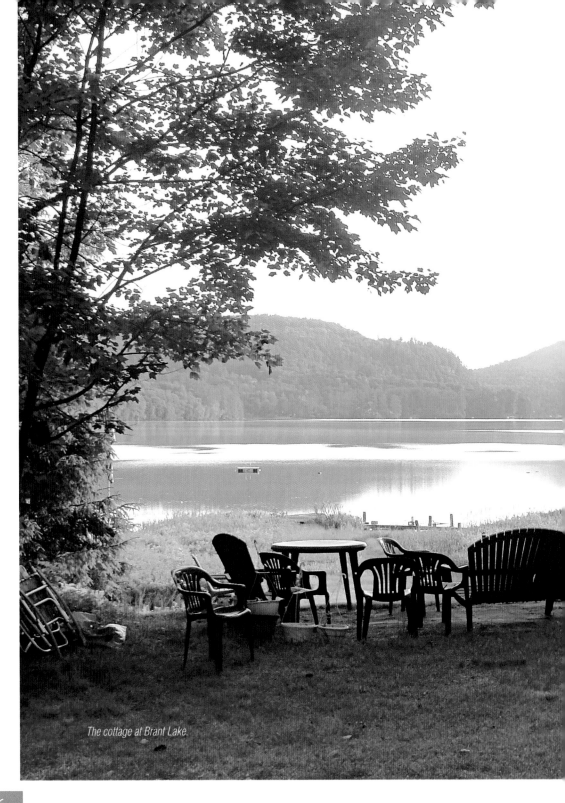

The cottage at Brant Lake.

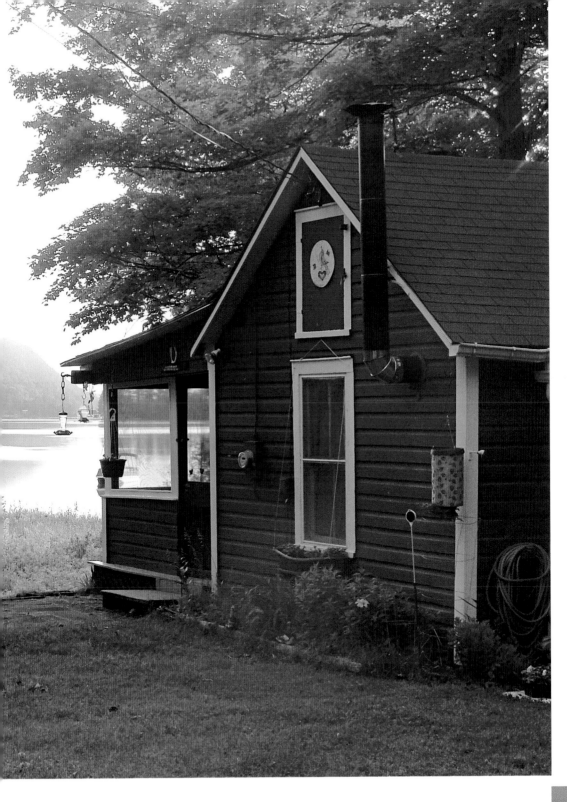

Dieting with my dog

legged barn table in the middle of the room. Kelly curled so tightly on a throw rug in front of the fire her nose touched her haunches. She hadn't slept so soundly in a long time. Her lips seemed to curve into a smile.

We'd been busy all day, touring the lake on the pontoon boat, exploring the tall grassy field at the water's edge, looking for bullfrogs from the dock. Kelly splashed along beside us, her belly dripping wet. We played Frisbee and threw sticks. Physical activity seemed natural here.

Unfortunately, so did food. Thick, smoky burgers seared with grill marks. Corn on the cob dripping with butter. Homemade creamy potato salad, none of which was on our healthy eating plan. But we were at the lake. This was vacation, calories didn't count. I'd gobbled down not one, but two cheeseburgers for dinner, and the feeding frenzy didn't stop there. After Nan and Pop had retired for the evening, Mike dealt the cards around the table for our traditional night-time game of Canasta. I scavenged through the kitchen cupboards.

"C'mon Peg," Mike called. Why was he so excited? After all, Andy had regularly trounced us at the game since he was eight years old. And we couldn't play games without a snack.

I opened the flame on the gas stove and settled an old cast iron pot on top. After adding a measure of oil and a handful of corn kernels, I covered the pot and smiled like a little kid. I enjoyed shaking the handle, waiting for the popping to commence. Microwaves took all the romance out of popcorn; you had to have active participation to feel the true satisfaction of the *poppity-pop-pop* sound as the kernels exploded.

When everything was ready I tipped the steaming treat into an enormous metal bowl, drizzled the corn generously with melted butter, added salt then took the bowl to the table.

Playing cards while munching on popcorn, I hardly noticed how often I plunged my hand into the bowl. The deep darkness outside the cabin windows, the sound of crickets singing, the stillness – this was not real life. This was

removed, a place where routines were broken, where the mundane patterns of life changed. Dieting rules did not apply here.

I tossed one kernel after another into my mouth. They were light as air. The practically weightless clouds couldn't possibly contain many calories – maybe they were even good for me! Kelly woke up and positioned herself at my feet. She was counting on a few kernels being dropped, and was soon rewarded.

"Two hundred basic, four hundred meld," I said, spreading out my cards, pleased with my score.

Andy laid down his hand. "Four canastas, two natural," he said. "Three red threes, a hundred points for going out …"

One thing I love about Canasta: the rules sound random, as if made up as you went along. Jokers and twos are wild, a deuce beats an ace, a red three is 100 points but a black three loses to all. You can draw off the discard pile one moment, but the next the pile is frozen. It feels like the players are talking a secret language, and every time we play I feel smugly smart.

As we continued playing, I noticed the dwindling level of popcorn in the serving dish. But I was the only one still eating. Repeatedly, I picked out the golden kernels and raised them to my mouth. Up, down, up, down; effortless exercise. Hunger clearly wasn't driving this repetitive motion, yet there was a powerful urge and pleasant reward with each puffy bite.

I continued blissfully munching until Mike moved the bowl to the other side of the table. Startled, I looked up and caught his expression. I froze. More than two decades of marriage had perfected my ability to read Mike's most subtle squint. His eyes narrowed, his lips tightened, his head cocked slightly to the side in a nearly imperceptible shake. "Do you really want to do this?" his expression asked.

Maybe he hadn't really meant it that way.

Looking for adventure at the waterfront.

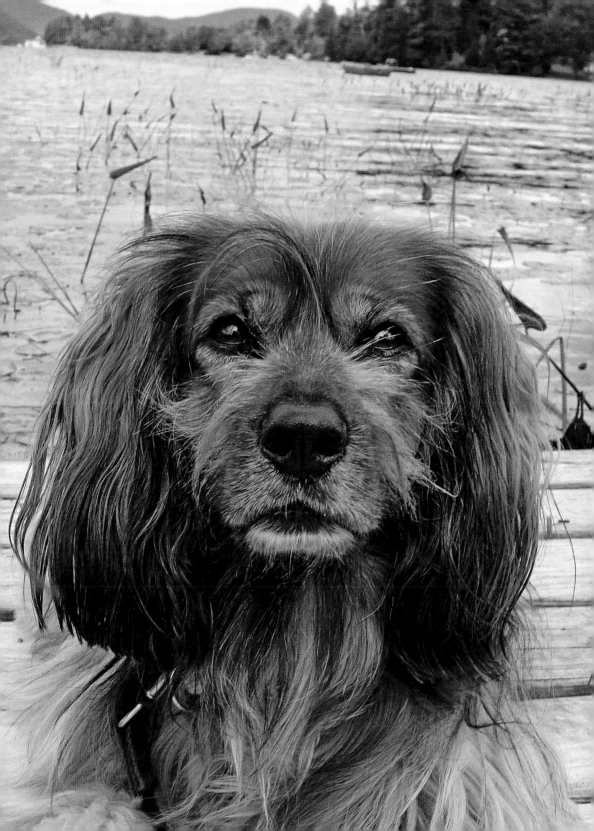

Dieting with my dog

Maybe he was just trying to help. I knew Mike loved me at any size. Maybe he was moving the bowl to keep it from his own reach. Nevertheless, the shame of all the times I'd been embarrassed by what I'd consumed resonated within me. The only defense for those painful feelings had been defiance. When asked, "You don't want to eat that, do you?" my spontaneous response was to get ready for a huge bite and reply, "Yes I do, and I will! Just watch me!"

I struggled to keep my emotions in perspective. *It's just popcorn. It's just this once.* We were there at the lake to have fun, weren't we? But Mike was right. I shouldn't have eaten all that popcorn, and I knew it. He'd controlled himself and I hadn't. *Now I'd blown my diet and ruined everything I'd worked so hard for.* I wiped my greasy fingers, wanting to throw the napkin over my face in shame.

That night I lay in bed, eyes wide open, clutching my belly, where the sweet, melting butter hardened into a sickening glop that cemented the popcorn, burger and potato salad into a bowling ball that rolled around, menacing my insides. Mike slept soundly beside me. Curse his popcorn-snacking restraint!

I hadn't felt this bad in months. I didn't feel like this when I ate healthy foods, or reasonable amounts. Was this worth it?

Years earlier, in young and foolish college days, I'd had the same realization after what I'd thought was a harmless evening at a party with friends. I didn't ordinarily drink, but that night I'd had a few beers – apparently a few too many – and crashed on my bed, fully clothed. The next morning the room was spinning. My stomach churned and my mouth felt like it was stuffed with cotton. Whatever had been fun about the evening before had long since ceased. I'd closed my eyes, but the room still spun. *This isn't worth it,* I'd told myself. And I meant it.

If only swearing off food was that easy for me. I could refrain from drinking, but I couldn't stop eating. One thing for sure, at that moment: over-eating wasn't worth feeling that sick.

I groaned quietly. Kelly stirred from her rug, padded over and jumped up onto the bed beside me. She licked my face. I liked to think I could sense when she was upset or lonely or sad, and it felt good to think that she could sense when I was hurting, too. She hovered over me like a mother whose child had flu. She was so calm, so gentle, nuzzling against me with simple devotion. This love was a reward far greater than the pleasure of anything tasty, delicious, appetizing, luscious or delectable. I stroked Kelly's neck as she curled up against my belly. Her body warmth instantly passed between us, and eased my aching stomach until I fell comfortably and soundly asleep.

How Kelly recognized my need for a dieting accomplice, I couldn't know. Had she sensed something that night as we curled together, the ache slowly dissipating from my body? Was it somehow an understanding beyond my own comprehension that compelled her to watch over me, like a furry conscience? From that night on, whenever I reached for a cookie in the kitchen she was there sitting on the floor, looking at me, her searching brown eyes beseeching me to stop and reconsider my actions.

Kelly already regularly sat by the front door, waiting for a walk. That made sense as she got something out of that. But now, she also padded in front of the elliptical machine, sniffing around at its base and pawing the long, narrow treads, then looking back at me on the couch. My dog had become my four-legged trainer.

One morning, after returning from our weekend at the lake, I frantically worked on deadlines at my computer in between trips to and from the basement with heavy baskets of laundry. That day I couldn't seem to concentrate on any of my tasks; putting away dishes in the kitchen, then moving to my office to check my email. Back in the kitchen, a loaf of hearty 7-grain bread on the pantry shelf caught my eye. Hmmm, I was getting hungry, and a turkey sandwich with curly green lettuce leaves and thick slabs of tomato would do the trick. Just as I raised my creation to my lips, the dryer timer shrilled. I set my lunch on the living room coffee table and dashed downstairs; folding the clothes while they were warm meant they'd stay wrinkle-free. It wasn't until I climbed back up the stairs and dropped the armful of fresh clothes onto the sofa that I suddenly remembered my canine-accessible lunch. Surely it would be devoured down to the last crumb as usual ...

Kelly sat right in front of the coffee table as expected, not three inches from my lunch, her eyes locked, unblinking, on my plate. Her muscles quivered but she didn't move, not even a whisker. I looked down, stunned. The sandwich was there, intact. Not even a corner of crust was gone.

I couldn't explain how but Kelly understood what I'd been trying to do and had joined me onboard the dieting bandwagon. Could a dog really learn self-control?

Wet nose, shiny coat

What was I doing, a few weeks after our trip to the lake, with chicken wing hot sauce dripping down my fingers, and a dozen bags of salty potato chips – and not even the baked variety – piled on my kitchen counter? Happily, I wasn't having a relapse, but simply being a good mom, preparing for Andy's high school graduation party.

I suppose the term 'good mom' was open to debate, however. Now that Mike and I were eating more wholesome food, I felt concerned about what Andy was eating. Sure, I could pack him oaty bagels for lunch, but chances were they'd end up in the trash can. He worked and earned his own money, and get-togethers with friends often involved fast food runs. I served a healthy dinner most nights, but convincing him to eat it was another story. Many evenings Andy wasn't even home for dinner anyway, but scarfing down sports drinks and cheese curls with the team on the way back from games.

And before I knew it, he'd be off to college. My influence at that point would be over!

Too bad we hadn't started eating healthily before, serving up fish, low-fat meals and fresh vegetables at dinner. I'd been apathetic about healthy food, and my only consolation was that although Kate had grown up with the same meals and snacks as Andy, as an adult, she ate salads, low fat yogurt and asparagus through choice.

Despite my earlier poor example, there was hope.

Andy had planned the menu for his graduation party. Chicken wings. Pizza. Fries. Onion rings. Chicken fingers. Chips. Mozzarella sticks. All teen staples. How could he live on this stuff? I'd always known they weren't exactly healthy, but now I mentally calculated just *how* unhealthy they were. Six wings had as many calories as 30 slices of the turkey breast Mike and I used on our sandwiches. And the fat content of all that food? Assuming an average person on a diet allowed themselves 24 grams of fat per day, just one large serving of fries or a handful of mozzarella sticks could more than double their daily intake. A celebratory paper plate full of each of Andy's favorite foods would supply roughly enough partially hydrogenated oils and trans fat to fill the Alaskan pipeline.

"How about I add a salad to the menu? At least for the adults." I'd asked.

"Whatever." (This amounted to agreement in teen-speak.)

I covered a full bowl of chicken wings in sauce to marinate while we were at the graduation ceremony. Reaching down into the refrigerator crisper, I selected some cucumbers for the bonus healthy salad. As I stood up, my head swam, and my vision darkened. I caught myself on the edge of the kitchen table. Maybe I was trying to do too much, too fast.

My emotions were catching up with me; I teared up every time I saw a commercial for Huggies, wondering what had happened to my little redheaded boy who'd toddled around the house in a diaper. Goodness! What would Andy say if he knew his mom was thinking about diapers on his graduation day?

Ignoring the dizzy spell, I marched upstairs to where Mike was getting ready for the ceremony. I slid into a new dress bought for the occasion – a simple, white and teal number with a mock-wrap top that emphasized the smallest parts of me and had a slimming waistline. The dress floated over my middle without clinging, and flowed away at the hips. I smoothed the skirt with a satisfied smile. This was the first time in a long while that my 'look' felt somewhat pulled together.

Mike adjusted his necktie in the mirror. "You look great," he said, taking in my reflection behind him.

"So do you," I replied. In addition to Kelly, Mike was benefiting from our new diet. My whole family was taking on a new shape, in more ways than one.

That afternoon Mike and I sat on mauve-cushioned chairs in the packed Gothic Revival chapel of Andy's school. Organ music floated down from a loft. I'd always loved the space here, the soaring arches naturally elevating my thoughts heavenward. We'd attended many ceremonies over the years, from academic award programs and solemn candlelit Christmas services, to school graduations as Kate and Andy progressed through the grades. This would be the last one for us.

I enjoyed the pageantry of the formal occasion. Maybe I was one of the few who took pleasure in lengthy speeches, and traditional songs – the ones you could count on year after year – caused my eyes to brim with tears. The only thing I didn't enjoy was having to get up and down so often. Stand to sing. Sit down.

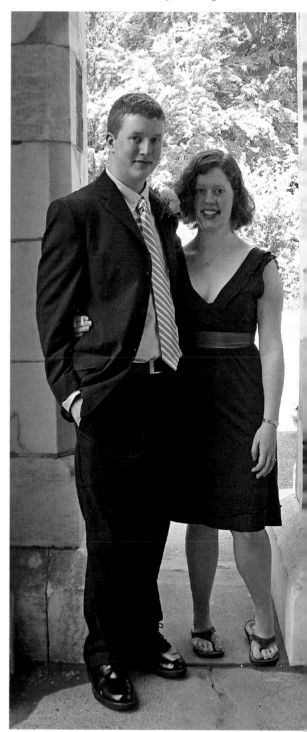

Andy and Kate (ages 16 and 20), ready to fly the nest.

Dieting with my dog

Stand up for this reading. You may be seated. The room wobbled after a half dozen times of this. My hand reached out to steady myself on the back of the seat in front of me. Another dizzy spell; I'd been pushing too hard.

After the speeches were read and hymns sung, the students began filing forward. Mike put his arm around my waist. Andy rose from his seat, tall and lean. He walked confidently to the podium, shook hands along the line of smiling academia and received his diploma. He'd graduated. With the very next step he was an adult. His journey away from home, away from me, had begun.

Mike and I cleared the navy and green paper plates from the table. The party had been a hit. Everyone loved the food, and there weren't any objections to its lack of nutritional value. I'd even eaten a slice of gooey pizza, without the urge to have another. Despite the enthusiasm, however, there were heaps of food left over.

"What are we going to do with all this?" I asked, packing messy chicken wings into plastic containers. Kelly joined us, her head following the food's journey from table to fridge. A runny residue at the bottom of the wings pan made me grimace. I wasn't tempted to cheat and snitch even one. The grease, which in the past marked the presence of something delicious, now signified instead something I wanted to stay away from.

"And this." Mike frowned, sliding pizza into a storage bag. Although we'd each enjoyed a slice at the party, we didn't want the leftovers to hang around. Amazingly, only a few short months ago we'd have been embracing the leftovers, giddy over the grease and pepperoni. I wrapped the pizza in foil. Kelly whined. It wasn't that we'd suddenly begun to hate pizza; I still considered it one of the most delicious foods ever created, and it even contained some redeeming ingredients: tomato sauce, veggies. We just saw

pizza more clearly, evaluating it and choosing to eat just one slice, make a healthier version, or skip it all together. Food wasn't controlling us any more. *We* were in control. I stacked the food in the fridge and closed the door, pushing tightly against it as if to prevent escape. Andy and his friends would enjoy most of the leftovers.

Congratulating myself, I turned away from the fridge, only to see Kelly contorted at my feet, her posture crooked. Her hind legs quivered. Her eyes darted. Kneeling to comfort her, I felt her whole body shake.

"Mike, something's wrong!"

He bent down and called to Kelly softly. She tentatively wagged her tail and, at first, I thought she was okay. But when she tried to walk to Mike, she fell over.

Her legs didn't work. She floundered across the cold tile floor, wobbling like a lopsided wind-up toy. "It's okay, Kelly," I said through a tight throat. Trying to remain calm, I stroked her legs. She quieted some, although the scary shaking still afflicted her little body. Even as she shuddered, her eyes looked up at me with deep trust – an expression that tore at my heart because I had no idea what to do to help her.

Three minutes later it was all over.

Later that night I was the one shaking. Terrifying thoughts of brain tumors and incurable diseases ran through my mind. I couldn't imagine life without Kelly. *God, please let her be okay.* One thing I knew for sure – Kelly depended on me to keep her healthy, and I wouldn't let her down.

The next day the vet, Dr Dietrich, listened to Kelly's heart and looked into her eyes. Mike stood beside me while I fidgeted in the chair. Kelly remained calm as the doctor gently rotated her limbs. It was as if nothing had happened.

"There could be several possibilities," the vet suggested, still prodding Kelly on the examining table. "Epilepsy, Cushing's disease."

I held my breath.

"We could do an MRI to look for any brain abnormalities. But to be honest, that is very expensive, and may not give us a definitive answer." She paused and studied Kelly's chart.

"Let's run some blood work first and see what that shows. We should get a CBC, thyroid profile, heartworm check …"

The vet instructed a technician to gather supplies from a cabinet.

"It sounds like she may have had a seizure. There may be environmental or nutritional issues."

My eyes brimmed with tears. Were we innocently poisoning Kelly? Maybe there was something in the house, carpet cleaner, air spray, something that had caused her seizure. The list could be endless. Or her food. We bought the best quality dog food we could afford. But maybe that wasn't good enough. Should we feed her organic? The raw diets I'd heard so much about? Homemade?

Our vet suggested it would be difficult to isolate a cause. "If it's epilepsy, the episodes could start happening more and more. It could be months or longer in between. Or it might never happen again. I suggest you make a record of any time she has an episode; what happened, how long it lasted. What happened right before the episode."

We nodded solemnly. Epilepsy sounded serious. I'd do anything to make sure Kelly was okay. Dr Dietrich encouraged us to watch her closely and call if we had any concerns.

Before we left, we led Kelly up onto the big scale. The digital numbers bounced around.

"Thirty-six," Mike announced. I smiled. She'd lost five pounds.

"Congratulations," Dr Dietrich said. "It's not easy to manage your dog's weight at home. You're doing a great job."

A few days later our vet called and gave us the encouraging news that Kelly's blood work was all negative. The diagnosis was idiopathic seizure; seizure with no identifiable cause. We'd do whatever it took to make healthy changes in Kelly's food and environment.

I started the symptoms notebook then tucked it away, hoping I'd never have to look at it again.

I had to take care of Kelly, she depended on me. I'd never let her down, but in order to fully care for her, I had to take care of myself, too. There was something I could ignore no longer.

The following week I sat on the paper-covered table in my doctor's office. "I've been having these dizzy spells," I explained. Thoughts of my cousin, Judy's, heart attack nipped at my mind. Had she mentioned vertigo as an early symptom? She'd said she was tired. I'd been feeling run down. Did I feel a pressure on my chest like she had? Maybe I wasn't having a heart attack yet, but it could be clogged arteries. Aneurism. I continued self-diagnosing as my doctor inflated the blood pressure cuff. With every squeeze on my arm, I imagined more and more serious illnesses.

"Well, what is it?" Mike asked when I returned to the waiting room. Over the last few weeks he'd noticed me lose my balance when I stood suddenly. His brow furrowed with concern.

I took my old bottle of blood pressure medicine out of my pocketbook. "Turns out, all my dieting and exercise have lowered my blood pressure enough. So taking pills, too, was actually causing my dizzy spells. I can throw these away now," I said with a triumphant grin. "I don't need to take them any more!"

The doctor had always warned me of the consequences of being overweight. My high blood pressure, high cholesterol, and high sugar levels could only lead to worse problems if I kept gaining. My new habits had proved I could turn things around.

Yeah, I still missed jam donuts and chocolate chip cookies a little. But eating well and becoming fit was not only keeping the doctor away … it was beginning to feel good, too!

Dog days of summer

"I'm going to wash the car," Mike called, dangling a bucket of sponges and sporting a huge smile. I watched from the back door as he turned on the hose. It seemed that guys always grinned when they were washing cars. I couldn't understand the attraction. The futility of it all annoyed me. Sure, those perfect little water beads would form across the hood, and the buffed chrome would shine like sparkling stars. The first time the car went out on the road, however, it would rip through a puddle and splash mud all over again.

Was that what was going to happen to me? I'd lost weight before. I'd worked hard to make my body look its best. But then, at some point the weight went back on, and all my efforts were splashed with mud.

Apparently, Mike didn't find car washing and waxing futile. Or maybe he just enjoyed the satisfaction of working hard and getting outside in the sun. I breathed in the warm air. Birds called from a shrub near the driveway. Kelly sat at my feet, fixing me with her best beseeching gaze. Everything around me suggested it was time to get out the door. I slipped on my flip flops, gathered a mountain of papers and took my work outside.

I plunked into a patio chair beside the lilac bush, tucked my feet up under me, and started reading my research texts. A tiny breeze rippled the pages.

Kelly scuttled around the fenced yard, tail up, ears bouncing. The paperwork lying on my lap seemed to mock me; everyone was active but me. This would not do.

I got up, setting a rock atop my work to keep it from blowing away. Kelly bounded over to me like a floppy toy. I picked up a stick and threw it to her. She ran after it, brought it back and we played keep-away.

The next time I reached down to pick up the stick, however, it moved. "Ack!"

It moved again. It wasn't the stick at all, but something long and sleek, partially hidden in the grass. In our urban neighborhood, the wildlife consists mostly of crows, squirrels, and maybe a fat old toad in the garden. I didn't expect to see anything larger than a wooly bear caterpillar making its way through my tiny yard, and this was no caterpillar.

"Snake!" I screamed. "Snaaaaaaaaake!" Perhaps I should love all God's creatures, but I have a problem with reptiles. Snakes are sneaky. They don't walk or run; they slither. Slithering is devious. Snakes, poisonous or not, had fangs, I was pretty sure.

I sprang up onto the lawn chair. Kelly ran over to investigate. "Get away!" I shrieked.

We lived far from western deserts and dangerous Rattlers, and nowhere near boggy rainforests. It was unlikely an Anaconda would appear and swallow me whole. I knew that most

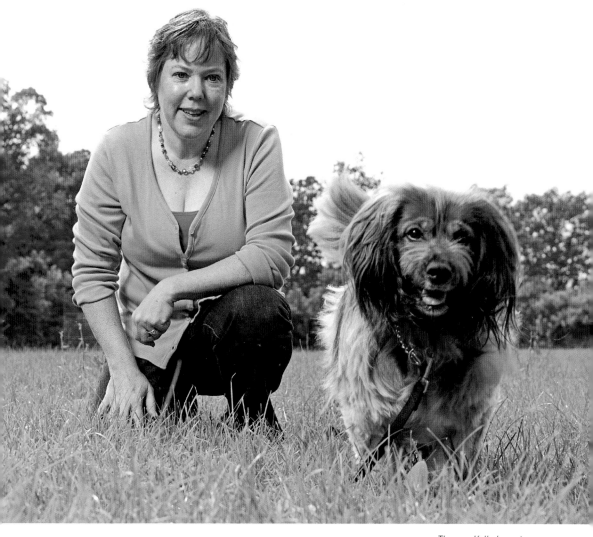

The new Kelly loves to run.

snakes inhabiting small northeastern cities were probably not poisonous, but I still didn't like 'em.

Mike dropped the hose and came running. "What? What?"

"A snake! Huge! About this long!" My arms spread about four feet apart.

"It's probably just a little garter snake," Mike laughed. "They won't hurt you."

"No. Those are green. This was brown. With stripes." My voice rose in fear.

By then, Andy had heard the commotion and appeared at the back door.

"Did it have long fangs, Mom?"

"Probably." I said, quite serious.

"And a little rattle at the end?" Andy shook his wrist mockingly.

"Look! Look, there it is!

I wasn't the only one who had noticed the movement in the grass. Kelly took an interest in the quizzical being which was now racing away, apparently to escape the sound of my bloodcurdling screams. Kelly pounced and scrambled after it.

What happened next was like a scene from

Dieting with my dog

a show on Animal Planet. Kelly had the snake in her mouth. She swung her head wildly, flinging the poor creature around like limp spaghetti. "No! Drop it! Nooooooo!" I yelled. "You'll get bitten."

"No she won't," said Mike. "that snake is only eight inches long."

Well, maybe it wasn't as long as I'd implied earlier, but it could still be dangerous.

Not wanting to approach too closely, I grabbed a rake and tried to poke at Kelly's side to get her to drop her prey. Finally, Mike marched over, placing his own life in peril, and grabbed hold of Kelly's collar. The snake fell to the ground in a tiny heap.

"I think it's dead," said Andy.

"It could be faking," I suggested.

Mike nudged the body with his sneaker. It didn't move. Kelly pulled against his grip, attempting to eat the remains.

"I think we've all learned a lesson here," Mike concluded, attempting to put the appropriate spin on the situation.

"That snakes are dangerous?" I asked.

"That Mom's crazy?" Andy responded.

Mike rolled his eyes. "Snakes are just something you're going to encounter outside. Nothing to be afraid of." He took the rake and scooped up the snake. Kelly ran off, excitement over.

"And Kelly's fine," he added, looking at me.

I consoled myself with the thought that plenty of exercise was available inside; a person didn't need to go outside with the fresh air and snakes in order to be physical.

My days consisted of cozying up to my keyboard with little chance of excitement. Periodically, I pulled Diet Cokes from the fridge, tossed a tennis ball to Kelly, and read some documents. True, my routine had been spiced up a little over the past few months: I took breaks to sweat on the elliptical; Kelly and I took walks. But, for the most part, I sat and worked. The biggest thrill I experienced was a foot cramp.

But I liked it that way.

When I was young, a sensible weight had been effortless to maintain. I'd eaten whatever I wanted without regard for calories or grams of fat. If my jeans felt a little snug, I just cut back on desserts over the weekend. As I got older I'd sometimes thought about calorie-counting, but for the first time, I now truly thought about when I ate, and why, and what was behind my habits. Fitness was a new concept, too. To lose weight, I had to burn more calories than I consumed. It would no longer do to shift between my desk chair and the living room couch. Turning the pages of a book could not be my most strenuous exercise. This was different, and new and surprising. And not so comfortable.

After the snake incident, I avoided lounging in the yard. I let Kelly outside, but refused to join her. When Kate called and said she'd be coming for a visit in a few weeks, I rejoiced and planned an assortment of indoor activities to do together. Kate enjoyed enclosed malls and movie theaters as much as me. Hurray!

One afternoon when I was Instant Messaging with Judy, I learned that she, too, had an unwelcome visitor. A snake had taken up residence under the stones on her front walk. She'd named the snake Sammy, hoping the familiarity would help alleviate her fear, but it hadn't worked. Her anxiety topped even mine. When I told her about the snake in our yard, she commiserated.

"So Sammy has a city cousin!" she exclaimed.

I'd been brave about the dogs running free in the neighborhood. I tried to take strength from that. But snakes right in my own back yard were a different story. That was where I drew the line.

I'd never seen a snake at my in-law's camp. Once Kate had reported seeing one gliding along beside her near the swimming float, but I hadn't actually witnessed this myself, so, for my own peace of mind, I refused to believe in its existence.

In late June we returned to the cabin for a mini-vacation. Kelly ran about, sniffing the air and poking into the chipmunk holes like always, making obvious her pleasure at being at camp. I followed her around at the end of the long leash, taking in the beautiful sparkling water beyond the sloping hill.

The quiet lake held little activity. No noisy jet skis or rowdy vacationers. A few fishing boats glided by; occasionally a sailboat with a bright red striped triangular sail. Children built sand castles on a beach in the distance. Years ago my kids had loved playing with their buckets and spades. In my mind's eye I pictured pre-school Kate in her blue-and-white striped bathing suit, uninhibited by her own three-year-old chubbiness. Andy, with a young, rollicking Hudson at his side, digging trenches to fill with water, maneuvering little plastic boats.

The years flipped past. I saw teenage Kate, in a bikini, laughing with friends, splashing each other and giggling. And Andy, walking toward the dock with his father and grandfather, taller than both of them, swinging a tackle box as he moved. I saw those years, and everything in-between, the memories floating across my mind in graceful progression. It felt good. The tension in my body melted, and a warm, gentle peace washed over me. Everyday life should be this relaxing, I mused.

I slid into a chair on the front porch with an iced tea and a captivating novel. The porch was wide and long, with tall, screened windows overlooking the lake. A row of rockers faced the view. I could have sat there all day and never tired of the scenery. Mike relaxed beside me, reading his newspapers. We exchanged a contented look. Kelly stood on her hind legs, looking outside. If nothing ever changed from that moment on, I'd have been content.

After the view, the next best thing about

sitting on those rockers was watching the activity at the big cylindrical bird feeder hanging from a limb right outside the windows. It attracted dozens of birds at a time, all colors; yellow finches, blue martins, red-winged blackbirds. The dining birds dropped plenty of seeds, drawing squirrels and chipmunks to the feast below. This was prime television for Kelly. She watched the animals intently, her ears cocked, her body quaking. Then, when she could stand it no longer, she let out a resounding 'woof' and sent the birds fluttering and the little critters scampering for cover. I imagined she felt quite powerful, havng that effect on so much wildlife.

That day, as we all watched, a gang of hungry ducks waddled up the hill and helped themselves to the scattered seed below the feeder. Kelly whined and trembled with excitement.

Andy appeared outside, causing the ducks

"There must be a chipmunk in here somewhere!"

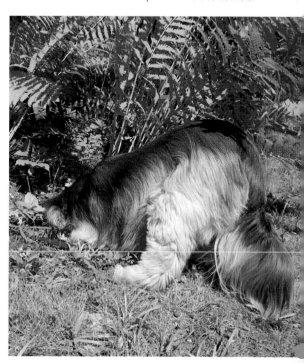

Dieting with my dog

to turn and skedaddle away. "Coming in!" he called, his arms full of spindly kindling for his grandparents' fireplace.

I moved to open the porch door. We always tried to get in and out quickly to avoid the company of pesky mosquitoes. But the wide load of twigs took some time to maneuver through, and Kelly chose that moment to make a dash for it. We usually took care that Kelly didn't slip out when the door opened, but the temptation of ducks in close proximity gave her lightning speed. Before any of us could react, she had bolted.

Knowing she ignored my calls under the best of circumstances, I held little hope of an easy return. I doubted I could outrun her, and in any case, she already had a substantial lead.

"Kelly, come!" I yelled, squeezing past Andy and the sticks and chasing after her.

She zig-zagged a crazy path after the ducks, heading toward the lake, which I felt was at least better than if she'd raced toward the road. As I ran after her, hollering futilely, I realized I'd neglected to grab her leash or some treats for bribery, or anything else that might prove helpful.

The ducks splashed into the water, Kelly close behind. She plunged in after them and paddled away.

"Kelly, come!" I continued calling, but she was so intent on the chase that she didn't even look my way. Kelly liked to swim, but she wasn't a strong swimmer, and usually just splashed around near the shore. "Kelllllly!" My voice rose to a frantic squeal as I hollered. I heard the porch door back at the camp thump closed and turned to see Mike and Andy running toward me.

Should I jump in after her? My long pants and sneakers wouldn't help me in the water, and my swimming skills were, well, poor at best. Besides, she'd now gone far beyond my comfort zone, swimming steadily toward the ducks as they glided deeper and deeper.

Mike and Andy piled into the rowboat. Andy undid the rope while Mike took the oars. They

seemed to move about a half an inch; rowing wasn't a speedy means of travel.

I was seriously concerned now. The lake was miles long, and a hearty swim across in width. Kelly was about at the mid-point when she paused and looked back at me. She knew she was in trouble.

"Kelly, come!" I called again. She looked at me, back at the ducks (now far from her reach), and back at me. Finally, she turned and tried to paddle my way. Her legs flailed and her head barely poked above the water.

Mike and Andy cleared the dock.

"She can't make it!" I shrieked. *What if she drowned?*

Kelly appeared to gasp as she struggled toward me. Her front legs splashed frantically. The rowboat neared, but she swam away from it. Fortunately, she wasn't moving fast.

Mike pulled up beside her and Andy grabbed her collar. He tried to pull her into the boat, but her struggling made it impossible to lift her heavy, wet body over the side. Stretching down, Andy held Kelly up while Mike rowed, guiding her toward shore.

I ran to the end of the dock and reached out. The water was over my head there, otherwise I would have jumped in, even in my clothes. As Kelly neared, her eyes fixed on me hopefully. It tore me apart how much she trusted me. My fingers grazed the ruff of her neck, found her collar and dragged her up onto the dock. She looked exhausted. But she was safe.

Back at camp, Kelly curled in the corner, put her face between her paws, and fell asleep.

"She certainly didn't have any fear, going after those ducks," my mother-in-law observed. "Not until she got in over her head. But she's fine now."

"Just had herself a big adventure," said Mike.

That's what happened when you put yourself out there into the world; you might end up with

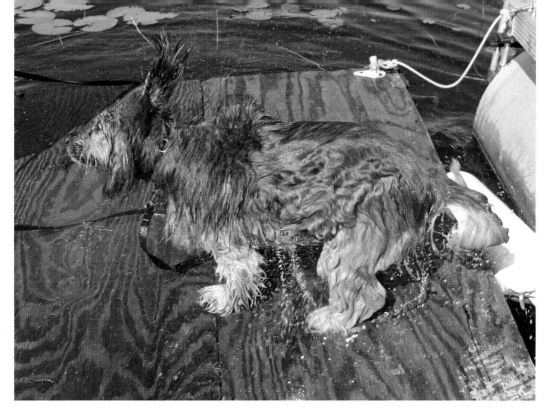
Shaking off a frightening experience.

a big adventure and get in over your head. The very thought made my palms sweat.

But it seemed that venturing out didn't have to be bad. Despite her scary struggle, Kelly seemed proud of herself, chasing after the ducks, unrestrained, going out deep into unfamiliar territory. When was the last time I'd gone for it, unrestrained? I usually held back, afraid of the unknown.

Getting out of the house and being active was my biggest challenge. Even at the lake, I preferred to relax on the porch and watch what went on, rather than joining in. Chasing ducks may be fun, but it could also put you in danger. Would Kelly have been better off staying safely inside? I watched her sleeping soundly, and smiled. Her paws twitched like she was dreaming. Maybe she was reliving her big adventure, in her dream actually reaching the ducks and scaring them away like the big, brave dog she was!

The next day Kelly raced around at the end of her long leash, exploring the woodpile beside some leafy ferns. I picked up a stick and threw it to her, then abruptly took off after it myself, enticing and teasing her with my chase. We fell to the ground and roughhoused in the grass, Kelly tossing her head and play-nipping at my sleeves. Maybe I'd get my shorts dirty. Maybe I'd get poked with a stick. Who cared? Lying on the grass, gazing up at the powder blue sky, a sense of fulfillment warmed me. It felt wonderful to use my body, every limb, to run and tumble. I turned and toppled along in the fresh greenness until my head hit a rock. I paused for a moment and rubbed the back of my neck. "Not so bad," I admitted, as Kelly and I continued rolling down the hill.

A pat on the head

Our New York climate offered only a brief window of opportunity for enjoyable outdoor activity. I'd begun my diet and exercise program months ago, in the winter, when snow flurries pelted me in the face and temperatures dipped like a donut in a coffee cup. Tugging on heavy boots and wrapping a scarf around my neck only to step outside and slip on the ice hadn't exactly thrilled me. Some days even Kelly shrank from the frosty air, and she wore a fur coat! Quick dashes around the block in the chill probably hadn't burned too many calories, but maybe my teeth chattering had helped work off a few more.

Now that spring had sprung, however, our walks were longer and more pleasant. The gentle warmth caressing my cheeks, and redolent gardens coming into flower made each outing a joy; a happy state of affairs that lasted for about three weeks. Then summer hit with a humidity that made a walk around the block feel like a day in the sauna. Kelly moved more slowly as she investigated the neighborhood. The city landscape wasn't nearly as thrilling as my in-laws' woodsy camp, but – to a dog – had an appeal all its own: old tom cats hiding under parked cars; overflowing garbage cans at the curb; fire hydrants; candy wrappers; cigarette butts. And you never knew what you might find in the storm drains.

I still walked with an eye out for loose dogs, but I didn't need to worry about pedestrians.

Kelly wanted to greet them all. More to the point, she begged for their attention. Her love of getting outside and walking partly stemmed from all the people she met who wanted to make a fuss of her. She didn't care if the man approaching us on the sidewalk hadn't even noticed her, or the teenager waiting at the bus stop was afraid of dogs. She'd still look up at their face and cock her ears, hoping for a pat on the head.

As we approached an intersection, she tried to move closer to a car that was waiting at the red light. I guided her back, whereupon she stood on her hind legs and peeked in the car window. The young woman in the passenger seat laughed and waved. "Cute!" she mouthed. Kelly seemed to smile. I walked with a spring as I held her leash. It felt good to be noticed; I felt like I'd received a pat on the head, too.

A little boy on a tricycle began to keep pace with us along the sidewalk. His babysitter watched from her front yard. "Doggy!" the boy said. Kelly sniffed at his chubby legs as he pumped the pedals. At least we could move as fast as a three-year old on a trike!

Around the corner, two young girls ran up to us. Kelly strained at the webbed lead, attempting to assault their faces with her tongue.

"She's big," the little girl sporting a pink t-shirt with red hearts giggled.

"Big?" I asked. By most standards Kelly was a small dog, medium at best. Big was a German

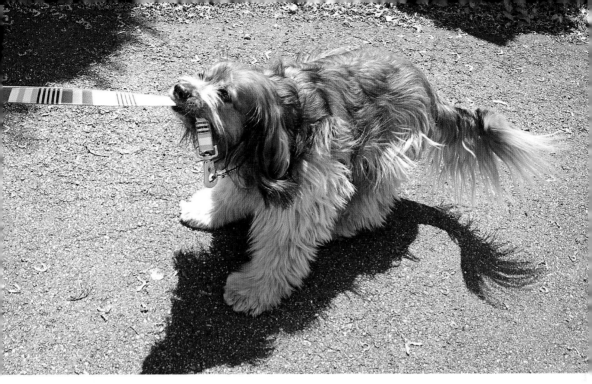

Kelly can't get enough of our walks.

Shepherd or Labrador Retriever. In comparison to a Toy Poodle or something similar, she was big. "Do you have a small dog at home?" I asked.

"No," the girl said. "We have a big dog, too."

Hmmm. Big? I looked down at Kelly. There was only one other thing the girl could mean, and it wasn't about height. Kelly had been losing weight along with me, but I wasn't sure how much. She'd been on the scale a few times since the first time I'd weighed her, but it was such a hassle we didn't repeat it often. I took a good look at her frolicking by the girls' feet. Maybe she wasn't doing as well as I'd thought. "Do you think she's fat?" I asked, afraid to hear the answer. Children are known for their honesty.

"No," the girl with the long pigtails replied, running her hands briskly across Kelly's back. "But her *fur* is fat."

The girl in pink nodded in agreement. I chuckled, relieved. Kelly's reddish-brown hair was long and unruly. It fluffed up at the sides and frolicked along her haunches. Her bushy limbs resembled miniature Clydesdale legs. Although her wooly shape seemed to indicate a chubby body, underneath she was much more compact. A good haircut would go a long way toward streamlining her new figure. I made a mental note to check with a groomer.

That Saturday Mike and I went out for lunch. A woman stopped me in the parking lot. "Peggy? Peggy, it is you! Have you lost weight?"

We had just stepped out of the healthy sandwich shop, which now replaced fast food burger and fry joints for quick meals. While we couldn't eat the same cheese and mayo-laden, foot-long sandwiches we used to enjoy, we could still find inexpensive and relatively filling selections with multi-grain buns, lean meats, and lots of veggies.

It took me a moment to recognize the woman as the mom of a girl Andy had known from nursery school. We used to gather with the other

Dieting with my dog

moms and dads to wait for our kids to finish singing the *Goodbye Song* and swarm toward the door. There in the hall, I'd shrink back behind her long, lean figure.

If we'd been schoolmates together, she'd be the popular, willowy basketball player and I'd be the team mascot. Tall people made me feel insignificant. Tall, lean people made me feel even worse. It didn't help that her blonde hair was expertly layered and highlighted. Mine was thin and shaggy, sprigging out like Kelly's wayward strands. Her khakis weren't frayed at the hem like mine, and they flowed over her hips snug and wrinkle-free, whereas mine looked like they'd rolled around inside a cement mixer. I couldn't imagine appearing so tidy and stylish. Who'd have guessed nursery school could make a person feel so inferior?

She tucked a lock of that perfect blonde hair behind her ear and smiled as we chatted and caught up with each other and the kids. Then she repeated her question. "You've lost weight, haven't you?"

"Well, yes I have," I admitted, feeling my cheeks flame, "a little." I'd weighed myself that morning, and actually it was more than a little. Thirty-six pounds to be exact. I still didn't quite believe it was true. To say it out loud felt like a lie – like when, as a newlywed, I'd been asked for my name. I loved my new surname, but it hadn't felt like mine. It didn't fit yet. The same was true of my new weight.

But my weight loss was hard to deny. When I stood up, my pants slid down. Shirts that had previously gaped open now hung loosely. I'd even unearthed the boxes in my closet and pulled out a few of the larger articles of discarded size twelve clothing. Cautiously, I'd pulled on a pair of jeans. They slid over my thighs and fastened comfortably at my waist. Actually, they were loose.

I could also see the weight loss in my face. Unlike a flabby tummy and massive upper arms, the face is one feature that can't be hidden by clothing. Looking in the mirror, I could see a hint of angular bone structure where chubby cheeks once bloomed. My chin was sharper. I actually had a neck. I recognized this girl!

"Have you lost weight?" was a question I was asked more and more often. Sometimes it was more tentative; "You look different. Did you get a new hairdo?" Sometimes it was assertive, "Wow, you dropped a ton!" I never knew how to take that one, since it implied that I'd been a tank before.

I wasn't offended, though. I *had* been heavier before, and I'd been working hard. If the results of my efforts were starting to show, then that was a positive. "Mike and I've been working out some," I now responded to the willowy basketball player, taking Mike's arm.

"Well, you look great," she said, nodding as she scanned my new figure. I straightened my shoulders. I wasn't quite as short compared to her as I'd thought.

Before we parted she glanced at my middle, then patted her own tiny tummy. "Guess I have to get back in gear and lose some of this." She walked off, slowly shaking her head.

Had this slender woman actually regarded me with even a twinge of envy? She was still tall and lean without any doubt. But did she actually feel insecure, like I used to when we waited in the nursery school hallway together?

"You look great, too!" I gushed loudly.

She turned, her brow furrowed for a moment, then broke into a wide grin and waved cheerily. "We'll have to get together again!" she called back.

Mike and I returned to the van. "You really do look great." He smiled as he held open the van door. "I'm proud of you." I knew Mike loved me fat or thin. He'd told me I looked beautiful when I felt the size of a cow. That beauty was perceived with a loving heart, not critical eyes. Hearing him say it now, though, I felt worthy of his appreciation.

The seasons had changed and, in the throes of summer, I was changing, too. I hadn't only shed the heavy outer wrappings of winter, but the weighty cloak of discontent and shame was also beginning to slip away. To have my efforts recognized, to be told that I looked good, made me want to run, jump up to the sun, and sing out loud right there in the parking lot – three impulses I'd never acted upon. Maybe I shouldn't need outside validation; my own feeling of accomplishment should be reward enough. But I couldn't deny it. The compliments felt good!

We hadn't seen Kate for nearly a year. I'd accepted that in my head, but not in my heart. The cell phone conversations helped ease my longing to hear her voice, and frequent emails and chats kept us up to date, but nothing replaced her hugs, or our shopping outings, or late night chat sessions in her room. And, hard to fathom why, but both Mike and Andy refused to help me paint my toenails ...

The time apart hadn't been a breeze for Kate, either. Sometimes I put her on speakerphone so she could join us in mundane activities such as grocery shopping and solving crossword puzzles. "It's Frezon family car ride!" she gushed one day as we engaged in a four-way cell conversation on the drive home from a game. Although she was busy, I could tell she felt left out when I talked about family birthday gatherings and trips to the lake.

So when she found herself with a free weekend over the Fourth of July holiday, and her husband was unable to get away from work, she booked a flight to come visit. Three days with us. Three full days to visit, face to face. We'd miss Aaron, but I also felt a secret delight at having my little family intact again, the way it used to be.

"I'm here!" Kate called from her cell phone after collecting her luggage. We drove up to the airport pick-up area just as she walked out to meet us. I barely waited for the van to slow before I flung open the door and ran to her.

While we hugged, crowds elbowed past us on the busy walkway. Rolling suitcases bumped into my legs. "I missed you!" I said above the distorted announcements blaring from the speakers. I knew we had to clear the way, but I didn't want to lose the moment. I had Kate back home again.

"Mom!" Kate threw her arms around me, noting how different the hug felt. "You've changed!"

Well, that was ironic; I'd spent so much time grumbling that my kids wouldn't stay the same and there I was making changes of my own. Some pretty major changes, too. Maybe staying the same wasn't always best. Sometimes change was necessary. Sometimes it was even good.

"Let's go," Kate said. Andy picked up her bags and loaded them into the van. I hopped into my seat and Kate piled in – a *real* Frezon family car ride! Even though at home things were different – and that was good – for three days I'd get back a little of our previous life together.

As she stepped in the door, Kate noticed right away the changes in the house. "There's an elliptical in the corner!" (definitely not a piece of furniture she'd ever expected to see in our home!).

"Wait 'til you see the kitchen." I showed her the cupboard which once held chips and cookies, now loaded with almonds, wheat crackers, and high fiber protein bars for snacks.

And the refrigerator stocked with fresh strawberries and romaine lettuce.

"No M&M's?" she teased.

"Just these," I showed her the special green *I Love Peg* M&M's. I'd put them in a small glass jar with a tight cover. I hadn't been tempted to devour a single one. They were love.

"Wow," she said.

Late that night I sat on the edge of Kate's bed, just like I used to. Sometimes, our bedtime talks had gone on for hours, the glow from a streetlight peeking in through a gap in the curtains. Just the two of us together, we shared happy moments and made big plans, revealing

Dieting with my dog

feelings that sometimes ran too deep to fully understand. I pulled the light comforter up around Kate's shoulders. "How does it feel to be back in your old bed?"

"Weird," she said.

I confess I was hoping for longing in her voice, but her reply reassured me. To feel weird to be back at home must mean she felt comfortable where she lived.

Kelly ambled into the room, jumped up on the bed and curled by my side.

"She can't be away from you for a minute," Kate said.

"She's checking up on me, making sure I'm not cheating on my diet," I laughed.

Kate grew quiet. "You've done really well," she said so softly that I had to lean closer to hear. Then, I saw the tears sliding down her cheeks.

"Kate – what?" I smoothed a stray red curl from her cheek and waited. Snuffles became sobs. I rubbed her back.

"I'm just … I'm sorry …" she sniffed.

"It's okay." Kate was my level-headed girl. She'd had disappointments and letdowns like everyone, but she always handled them well. She was rarely whiney or dramatic. Usually, I understood her emotions, but this time I was struggling. Had something happened at home? Maybe she and Aaron had had a fight?

"I'm being dumb." She lowered her eyes apologetically.

"Ha," I said, "I know that feeling. You're in good company."

"No, Mom." She wiped her eye with the tip of her forefinger. "I'm proud of you. Really. But seeing you so skinny … don't take this wrong, but it sorta makes me feel bad about myself. I've never seen you like this, and, well … I'm so embarrassed that I haven't made enough effort myself …"

"Oh, Kate!" I held her close and her tears started afresh.

Kate had gained a few pounds, going up a dress size or so in the past few years. According to the charts, she was maybe a handful of pounds off the ideal weight, but to me she looked just about right. Of course, it hadn't helped that she'd grown up in a household with a poor example of diet and physical fitness. She shared my weakness for sweets. Mike always said there was nothing more frightening than watching Kate and I share a dessert; like two lions tearing into their prey, each one determined to get their fair share. As a teen, she wasn't stick-thin with a perfectly flat midriff like some of her classmates, but that never caused her to go on a starvation diet, or make voodoo dolls of all her skinny friends. I always felt she had a healthy body image.

"You're not fat," I said.

"Well, I have gained a few pounds since getting married," she said. "We go out to eat a lot. I'm sitting at my desk job all day instead of getting exercise walking all over campus. My clothes aren't fitting the same … my pants are kind of tight. I … I just didn't want to admit it."

"It's natural." I kissed her wet cheek. "You're older, your daily routine changed. You look just fine. But if you're unhappy, you can adjust. Listen, if I can do it, you can, too! It wouldn't take much to cut back a little here and there. Take a walk after work. Things like that."

"You're right," she said, sniffing. "I know. I just didn't want to accept it."

"Lots of things change that we don't want to accept," I said. "But they usually end up okay."

Kate leaned over and gave me a hug. "You look wonderful," she said. "You really do. I'm proud of you."

"I'm proud of you. too," I said. And I was.

After our goodnights I turned off the light and Kelly followed me out of the room. I leaned down and ran my hand over her back. She really was slimmer under all that bushy hair. "I'm proud of you, too," I said, patting her on the head. She slurped my face in thanks.

Dogcessories

"Time to get all beautiful," I said, leading Kelly into the grooming salon. She wagged her tail and high-stepped happily. This was the reward for all her hard work, the haircut that would help show off her new svelte canine figure.

However, the moment I handed the leash to the groomer, Kelly howled like she was being abandoned in the woods. I knew Kelly was attached to me, but hadn't realized she could exhibit such major separation anxiety. I tried to leave, but the pitiful noise made me stop and turn; I couldn't walk out on her.

The young woman in the pawprint apron grasped the leash, but Kelly pulled it out of her hand and leapt, clearing the low swinging door that separated the work area from the reception room. She clawed at my leg desperately.

"Uh … can I just stay?" I asked.

The groomer shook her head. "Sorry. We find it distracting to the dogs."

I knew Kelly. She didn't like to be left alone, was upset by strange places, and nervous around other dogs. I'd already made arrangements to arrive at the parlor's quietest time to avoid as much stress as possible for Kelly, and paid extra for speedy treatment so she wouldn't have to be left in a cage. I'd done all I could to make her visit as comfortable as possible, hoping that maybe she'd even enjoy her girl's day at the spa.

But if this was the way she felt now, my leaving wouldn't help matters. "I think she'd be better if I stayed."

"Oh, they usually calm down the instant Mommy leaves," the girl assured me, swinging through the door and retrieving her client. "Don't you worry, we have your cell number on the paperwork if we need anything."

I sighed and gave Kelly an encouraging hug, then reluctantly headed out the door before I could change my mind. A look over my shoulder showed that Kelly was straining after me. I felt like a mom abandoning her child to the evil witch in the gingerbread house in the woods.

"Try not to baby her so much," said Mike. We'd stopped at the nearby grocery store while waiting for Kelly's transformation. "She'll be okay." His comment hit home as I'd been guilty of babying not only Kelly, but Kate and Andy, too. When they were little, I'd dropped them off at nursery school or play dates, then clung too long, worried how they'd manage without me. Sending off those signals, no wonder they felt stressed about parting from me.

Had I done the same now with Kelly?

We grabbed a shopping cart and began picking up provisions for our Fourth of July picnic later that day. Andy – who'd perfected the teenager weekend schedule of staying up into the wee hours – was home asleep. Kate was preparing a new salad she'd learned to make

Dieting with my dog

with spinach, fresh strawberries, and vinaigrette dressing.

Mike and I glided through the aisles, confidently filling the basket with healthy food. I didn't even think about the traditional hot dogs, potato salad and ice cream for our celebration. Actually, instead of the menu, I was thinking more about my family and the fun we'd have being together. Somehow, celebrating had stopped being just about the food.

As I was thumping the side of a heavy watermelon to test for ripeness, my cell rang.

"I think maybe you should come back," stammered the voice on the other end. "There's, umm, a little problem with Kelly."

"Kelly," I whispered to Mike, dropping the watermelon in the bin and abandoning the cart.

"Is she okay? What happened?"

"Well, she didn't like the bath, and she didn't like the blow dryer." There was a pause. "Her eyes are really, really red and … she's pretty stressed out …"

"We'll be right there."

When we arrived, Kelly nearly burst through the swinging door to get to us. She was wet and bedraggled, with tufts of hair sticking out all over. She panted heavily. My shirt became soaked as she tried to crawl into my lap. I felt her heart rate rising.

"I think she's burst the blood vessels in her eyes …" the girl said.

My education was lacking on the subject of burst blood vessels. I didn't think it was an emergency, but it shouldn't have happened. I took Kelly's chin and looked into her eyes. I gasped; they were as red as two cherries.

Mike shook his head. "How could you have let her get to this point? It's been two hours – why didn't you call us earlier?"

"Well, uh …"

The young groomer apologized as we quickly led Kelly away. Her scraggly mess of a coat couldn't have been a good advertisement for the grooming services as we marched out the shop.

I thought Kelly would relax once we got to the van, but she jerked and struggled uneasily. Then she slumped against me and gasped for breath.

"We're going right to the vet's." Mike hit the gas. Luckily, the offices were open on the holiday.

A check-up concluded that Kelly had burst blood vessels, a scratch on the eye, and an elevated heart rate, but she was going to be fine. The burst blood vessels had been caused by stress. The scratch must have happened somehow when she struggled against the bath or blow dryer. I hugged Kelly tight, my heart aching to think she'd been forced to endure something that made her so terrified, and all alone, too. The vet gave us antibiotics and eye cream, and we made an appointment to have her rechecked in a few weeks.

Back home, Kelly curled on her pillow. Kate could hardly look at Kelly's cherry red eyes, but Andy thought they looked cool.

"You tried to get beautiful and this is what happens." I gently combed her dried, tangled fur. Later, she napped as we picnicked in the back yard.

Fortunately, Kelly wasn't bothered by loud noises. At dusk she woke refreshed and ready to join us at the park for fireworks. She lunged for the door.

"Come on!" I called. "We're ready!"

I was zipping my favorite denim shorts when Kate appeared. "We've got to get you some new clothes," she said. "Those are so baggy they're falling off you."

"Are they really so bad?"

"Yup!" Andy said, joining us. While Kate might have been more tactful, Andy held nothing back. He'd recently teased that Mike's favorite sweater vest with the big brown buttons made him look like a dorky old man, and my rainbow-striped ribbon belt should be returned to the child I took it from.

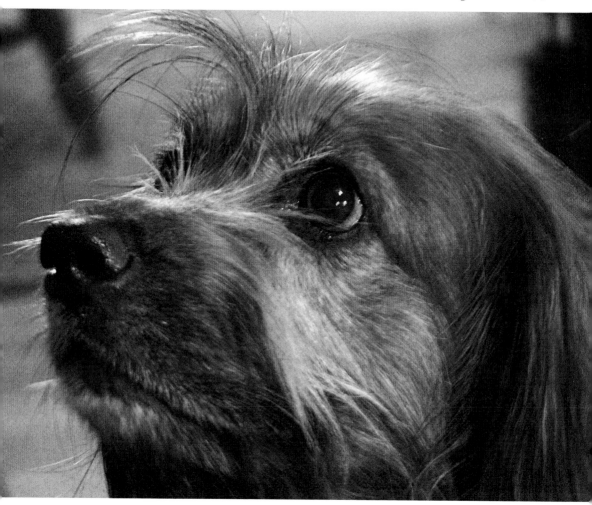

The vet helped heal Kelly's eye injury.

"What do you think, Mike?" I asked, motioning dramatically.

He held up his hands and backed away. He'd learned to stay out of these types of debate.

We walked in a group to the park; Kate and Andy in front, Mike linking my arm as I led Kelly, who trotted obediently by my side. I felt curiously invisible behind the kids, quietly observing them, eavesdropping on their conversation. These two were strangers, mysteriously unrelated to the curly, redheaded tots who used to race down the slides at the park. When we crossed the street I actually started to grab for their hands, then pretended to untangle Kelly's leash instead so they wouldn't notice.

The sidewalks filled with other families, babies in strollers, sleepy toddlers who would likely start screaming at the first loud firework. With relief, I realized I wouldn't need to worry

Dieting with my dog

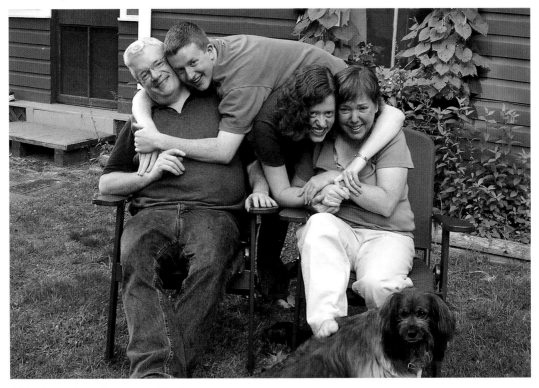

All together again, and having a great time!

about that, or nap schedules, or keeping track of little ones in the crowd. Maybe, one day the reverse would be true, and my kids would have to start taking care of me. Fair was fair.

I spread out the quilt and we huddled together. Kelly pushed her way to the middle. "Kelly, get off my feet," Andy complained.

"Well, if your big feet weren't taking up the whole blanket …" Kate teased. Some things never changed.

As soon as darkness settled over us, a rumble of loud pops erupted and the crowd cheered. I nestled close to Mike and he put his arm around me. Kate leaned into my other side and Andy sprawled across in front of us.

I lightly rested my fingertips on his shoulder. At that moment everything was perfect. Right then, I could reach out and touch each member of my family. The emotion of that thought filled me as a firework exploded overhead, brilliant green and blue sparkling side by side, expanding, then fading to darkness once more. I heard nothing. There was only the warmth, the feeling of perfect unity, and the brilliant color showering down around us.

Soon, sound returned, a powerful crack resounding, then echoing as it faded. But for that moment, there was only love.

Four explosions blossomed, one on top of the other. "Oooooooh," gasped the crowd.

One Fourth of July when Kate and Andy were very young, we'd listened to a family next to us naming the fireworks after their kids. At each colorful burst of light, the kids excitedly called out their name, claiming it as their own. Every year since then my family remembered this, and repeated those names as the best fireworks exploded. Now, as a brilliant gold rocket spread out into the most impressive sunburst I'd ever seen, filling the sky and sparkling in shimmering twinkles, my kids turned and looked at each other.

"Joshua!" Andy called.

"Emily!" Kate added, laughing.

It was a perfect Fourth of July.

The next morning Kate and I strolled together through the wide mall aisles. On Kate's last day home, she wanted to help me choose clothes to suit my new figure. "Forty pounds deserves a new wardrobe," she said.

"Well, maybe a few things." I'd reached the bottom of the last box tucked away in the closet, and had to admit, even those tops and shorts were too big. I hadn't weighed this little for twenty years. I'd been slim for a short while when Kate was around a year old. I'd long since given away the clothes I wore then, despairing of ever getting into them again. After that, my dress size had only increased.

As much as I'd loved having my whole family together the night before, it was also special having Kate all to myself. We laughed and talked as we roamed the mall halls. She was a skillful shopper, and while I usually stuck to discount department stores, afraid of the prices in the trendy shops, Kate knew how to find bargains in quality stores. "You like to wear jeans," she said, "so let's try Gap."

We scoured the racks in the back of the store and discovered several pairs on sale that looked promising. I took a size ten into the dressing room. I'd been under the impression that my baggy clothes made me appear slimmer. One look in the mirror, however, told me otherwise; they actually just looked like they didn't fit me. I slid on the new jeans, fastened the button, and stepped out to model for Kate.

"They look nice!" she said, inspecting.

"Actually, you might be able to go down a size. The butt's kind of baggy."

"Not a chance," I scoffed, trying to get a rear view. "The last jeans I bought were 18s. There's no way I could be less than a size ten now."

We'd been to several stores and tried on numerous styles, but the right fit eluded me. Either the seat was too loose, or my belly spilled over the waistband.

"Try these," Kate said, handing a different pair of jeans in through the curtain.

I tugged them on and stepped out for her to see.

"How do they feel?" she asked.

"They feel good. How do they look?"

"Great! You should buy them."

"I think I will." Back in the dressing room, I removed the jeans and took a look at the tag. "Kate!" I gasped. "They're a size eight!"

"I know!" she peeked into the dressing room, grinning.

"And they fit!" I squealed.

"I know!"

"They're an eight and they fit," I repeated, shaking my head. I folded the jeans over my arm and strode to the checkout counter.

"How about lunch?" I asked as I paid for my purchases. "There's a great salad bar downstairs."

"Okay," Kate nodded happily. "And then we'll shop for accessories. You'll need some shoes and maybe a necklace to finish off your new look."

I took her arm and stepped out of the store, feeling light as a paper airplane drifting in the spring breeze.

That evening I held up every new article of clothing to show Mike, then spread them all out across Kate's bed as she snuggled down to sleep for her last night at home with us. "Look at this one," I said, holding up a teal short-sleeved tee that appeared more Kate's size than mine.

"I know, I picked it out," she said cheerily.

"I'm going to try it on again!" I ducked into my room and returned wearing the teal top, and

Dieting with my dog

the new jeans. I stood in front of the full-length mirror on the closet door.

"You look fantastic, Mom," Kate said, without a trace of despondency about her own image. Only happiness, for me.

I turned, examining every angle. Although the reflection appeared different from months before, instead of seeing a stranger, I felt more like someone from long ago, the person I'd always thought existed under all the fat and baggy clothes. "I remember you," I said into the mirror. "You've been gone for a long time." I ran my hand over my trim tummy. "Welcome back."

Kate left the next morning. I hugged her goodbye, knowing that I had to let her leave again. My arms parted a little easier this time. Seeing her in one piece, happy and capable, I knew she'd be fine. And me? This whole flying the nest business didn't mean I was left with nothing. I had a fulfilling job, good friends, and a little dog who tagged around after me and licked my toes. A husband who loved me. And two kids we'd raised to be happy, successful and independent.

I'd changed. Kate had changed. My family had changed.

But it was okay.

A huge white van pulled into our driveway. The side panel depicted a stylized illustration of a pooch with a red bow and the word "Trans*FUR*mations."

"Now it's your turn, Kelly." She was finally going to get her haircut. Hoping this would be a positive transformation, I led her outside on her leash.

A woman in a zebra print coat and fur-covered pants emerged to greet us. I smiled as she fussed over Kelly, easily winning her trust. "Okay," she said, "shall we give you a new hairdo?"

The van was actually a fully-equipped mobile pet spa designed for convenient door-to-door

grooming. Melissa, the owner, had started the business for those who were too busy or unable to take their pets out to a grooming salon. She soon found her special niche in helping senior and fearful pets. We were in good hands.

There were no rules about dog parents having to leave; in fact I was welcomed inside. The interior was neatly arranged, with everything handily within reach. A noisy but functional air conditioner emitted blissful cooling air across the stuffy, confined space. Kelly hesitated, but followed me into the grooming van.

It took a bit more convincing to finally wrestle her into the tub. I tried to help keep her still as Melissa sprayed a gentle stream of water across her back and under her belly. When Kelly barked and nipped at the stream of water, Melissa didn't even flinch. She just laughed and continued the bathing. Although Kelly wasn't the most willing participant, she wasn't stressed out. Even the blow dryer, set at the lowest setting so as not to frighten, didn't bother her much. Once in a while she just nipped at the air coming out of the hose.

"Sorry," I said.

"Nah, it's a common reaction," Melissa, confidently wielding the dryer and a brush, replied. "She doesn't mean any harm, do you girl?" Kelly responded with a kiss.

My tension eased, knowing this groomer was in tune with dogs and their behavior. As well as she managed difficult temperaments, Melissa wielded the clippers with equal skill. Kelly relaxed once the drier was off, and let her paws be handled so that her belly could be shaved. Melissa even clipped Kelly's toenails quickly – *snip, snip, snip!* – something that usually took us nearly an hour to accomplish.

"This is great," I observed, watching an actual dog emerge from under all that scraggly fur.

A successful makeover by Melissa.

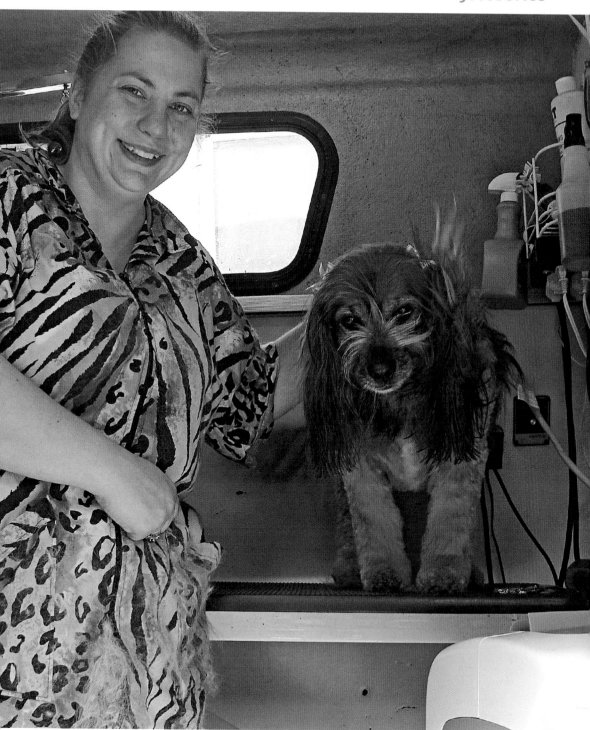

Dieting with my dog

When the job was done, Melissa squirted Kelly with doggy perfume and fixed light blue ribbons atop each long, furry ear, completing an excellent job of pooch pampering. I can't say that Kelly relished the treatment, as she bolted for the door, but she did put up with it, and at times even relaxed a little. And she looked fantastic.

"Thank you so much, I can't wait to show everyone!" I took care of the bill and promised to have the mobile spa return again.

Inside, Kelly pranced around the house, seemingly pleased with her new style.

"She looks great," Mike said.

"Yeah, Kelly, you're skinny," Andy observed.

New clothes. A new hairdo. I stooped to adjust Kelly's cute ribbons. Some fancy accessories. They weren't necessary, but a little pampering never hurt. Taking care to fuss with hair and clothes once in awhile were just the things to complete the transformation and make a girl feel good!

Like chasing my tail

In a few short weeks, Andy would be moving into his college dorm. Filling out forms, packing clothes and numerous other preparations took precedence over contemplation about what it would be like at home without him.

I'd been prodding and pestering for half the summer, asking him what he wanted to take with him. Planning wasn't his strong suit; baseball, summer job and friends were more on his mind.

Now we couldn't put it off any longer. It was time for a major shopping trip.

The morning was so hot that the walk down the hall felt like a stroll across the equator. If I could have sweated away the rest of my weight, the heat wave would have been welcome. Ordinarily, our summer temperatures hit the seventies or eighties, but that day it was approaching the high nineties.

Lately, the scale had become my nemesis.

Every morning I hoped it would show that the last chunk of unwanted weight had disappeared, yet every morning it refused to comply. I battled with the same few extra pounds for weeks, and every day I knew exactly which way things would go, too. If I'd indulged a bit too much – even in the healthier stuff that was mainly my food of choice – the reading was higher. If I'd been faithful about walking Kelly and sweating on the elliptical, it rewarded me with a lower figure.

Back and forth, up and down.

Although I'd made the simple cause-and-effect correlation, I continued playing the game.

Most distressing of all, my clothes had shrunk.

Okay, so that wasn't exactly true.

I stepped into the new plaid shorts I'd purchased as a reward and tugged the button through the buttonhole but – *ugh!* – the waistband squeezed me around the middle like a steer lassoed in a rodeo. These shorts hadn't even been through the wash yet, so I was hard-pressed to blame the dryer.

My belly muffin-topped over the waistband: not a pretty sight. I stomped to my bedroom, ripped off the shorts and tried a cute pair of capris. They fit, but wearing them and breathing at the same time would be a challenge. A second pair of shorts: also too tight. I kicked the discarded mass into a pile and slid into my trusty old elastic waist athletic pants. They'd never failed me.

In a way, I guess this was a positive; I knew my body now, and the way what I ate and what I did affected it. This was something I'd never fully considered before. Sure, I'd understood the basic principle of calorie intake and energy burned, but had never dissected my everyday actions in connection with this. Remaining out of tune with my body had made it easier to deny the problem.

I stood in front of the mirror and pulled on

Dieting with my dog

a light green tee. I'd always had trouble viewing my body objectively, because my mood and confidence determined what I saw, rather than what the mirror reflected. Sometimes, my gaze skimmed over my trouble areas, refusing to take in the bulges – surprisingly, at my heaviest, my reflection often revealed someone deceptively slim. Other times, I focused only on my middle, seeing only a beach ball with arms and legs. These two impressions could be just days apart. Did I actually know the *real* Peggy?

Looking at my body honestly, it was clear that, despite all the weight I'd lost, my stomach still wasn't flat, and love handles graced my sides. My accomplishments more than delighted me, but I wasn't skinny. At least ten stubborn pounds still clung to my frame, and even if they disappeared, there'd be no gorgeous long and lithe magazine model body in my future. I ran my hands down my curvy sides and scrutinized myself in the mirror. These days I saw what was truly there. A woman who had lost a lot of weight, who still had more to go, who would probably never be perfect, but who didn't have to be flawless.

Could it be I'd finally learned to accept myself as I was?

Acceptance, however, didn't mean I'd grown to love those last few stubborn pounds that clung to my middle.

I stomped into Kate's room and flung the pile of useless shorts into the dark closet. They fell at the base of a cardboard box, one of the very boxes that used to hold my 'fat' clothes. I'd worked so hard to empty those boxes; I couldn't start a new one all over again. Somehow, I had to figure out how to keep this weight loss going.

Returning to my room, I did what I always did when I had no answers. I offered up a prayer.

"Please, God, show me what I'm missing here."

"Hey, Mom?" Andy hovered somewhere in the hall outside my room as I strapped on my sandals. He always approached my bedroom cautiously and announced his arrival; even a show of maternal midriff was enough to scar his delicate teenage psyche.

"Do I have to go?" he asked, appearing gradually in the doorway – foot first, torso next, then face with downcast eyes last, just in case.

"Don't you want to help pick out your own supplies?"

"I don't think so. I don't really have a thing for sheets and matching towels and stuff."

That was obvious. Whatever towel Andy used for his shower was undoubtedly the one he found somewhere in the pile of clothes littering his bedroom floor. And if Andy even knew he had sheets on his bed, much less what color they were, I'd have been shocked.

I lowered my voice and sighed. "Would it be okay if we spent a little time together before you go away?"

There was a pause as he considered his options. "Okay, Mom," he said, defeated.

"We'll go out to eat after," I added, hoping to add an enticing bonus. Food he craved but could no longer get at home would be a perk. Few of my diet-friendly meals appealed to Andy. He'd nibble a small serving of the nutritious dinner served at the table, then be hungry again and make a late-night snack of frozen pizza, macaroni dinner from a box, or grilled cheese sandwiches. We weren't bringing home pizza and wings, or stopping for burgers anymore, but he still found them irresistible.

Before we left, I let Kelly outside for a quick run. The heat poured in the open doorway. "No walk today, Kelly," I said, "you'd melt into a puddle." We didn't have air conditioning in our old house, so I left a fan going to keep her comfortable. I filled her water bowl and tossed her a baby carrot.

At the department store, I pushed a shopping cart to the section piled high with home decor in bright colors and fanciful designs. The sign above read 'College 101.' Andy lagged a few paces behind. The stackable crates, erasable whiteboards – all the college bits and pieces filled my view, and all I could think about was

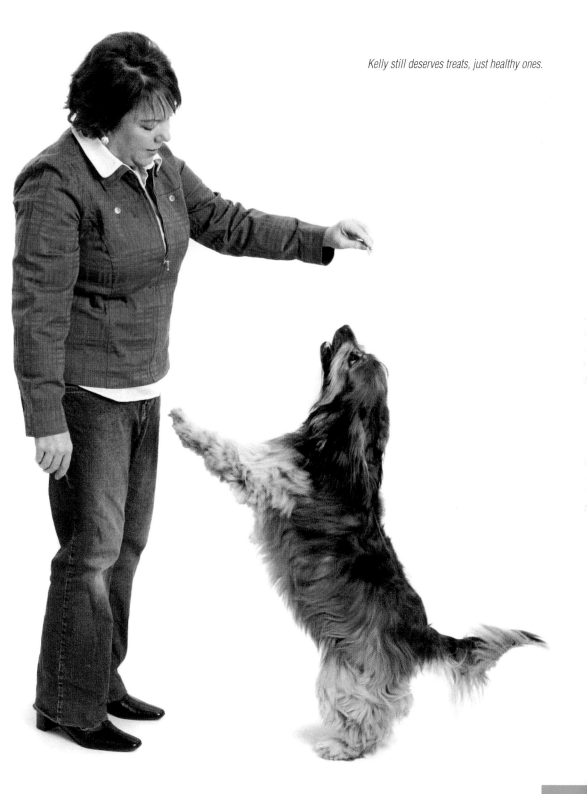

Kelly still deserves treats, just healthy ones.

Dieting with my dog

that the time had come for Andy to leave home. I rebuked myself sternly; we were there to get college supplies, not fret about my empty nest. I surveyed shelves of mattress pads and bedding thoughtfully. "What color sheets?" I asked, holding up a navy, a brown, and a black.

"There's a difference?" he asked, viewing the sheets from across the aisle.

"Cotton or jersey? Or flannel?"

"Whatever I'm using now is fine."

"Well, jersey is soft."

"Okay."

"But I think cotton is better."

"Fine."

"Maybe we should consider ..."

"Mom." His voice rose. "It's fine."

"You sure?"

"Cotton," he said.

I tossed the navy cotton sheets into the basket and grabbed a matching comforter. Andy declined to sample the texture of the towels, and was neutral about the under-the-bed box, though did take an interest in choosing some shelving units and a cool metal desk organizer. I ticked off supplies from a list. After notebooks, highlighters and a few other items, we were almost ready to go.

"Can you think of anything else?" I asked.

"A mini fridge with a keg?" he teased.

"How about socks? Boxers?"

"*Maw-ahm.*" Two syllables. "I've got socks and boxers." His cheeks reddened.

"Anything else you need?"

"Nah."

"A nice pillow? Poster?"

"Nah."

"A new desk light? Yours is kind of wobbly."

"It's not wobbly."

"Anything ...?"

Andy rolled his eyes and backed away. Whenever things felt tense, I got pushy. Letting go gracefully was going to take a little more work.

We headed toward the checkout. "Thanks, Ma," Andy said, glancing sideways.

"Let's do lunch," I said. We didn't go out together often, and I was going to enjoy it.

Later that night the three of us sat in the living room, still trying to get comfortable in the heat. The late night hour hadn't brought any cooling drop of temperature. Mike and Andy watched a baseball game on television. I worked at the computer. Every fan in the house whirled – the ceiling fan, a floor fan, a window fan across from my desk.

Suddenly, everything came to a standstill. The lights flicked off. With an audible whirr fading like a slide whistle, the television went dark and the computer shut down.

"Power outage. I'll get the flashlights." Mike felt his way through the darkness to the kitchen drawer. He peered out the window down the darkened street. "Everyone's out." Even the streetlights were off.

"It's hot," Andy said. With the fans off it had taken only a second for the stifling heat to fill the room. Mike opened the doors, but there was no breeze.

We waited, staring at the blank television the way Kelly sometimes stared at her empty supper dish, thinking food would magically appear.

I couldn't concentrate on reading with only a dim flashlight beam.

"Yeah, it's hot," I said, conversational agility evaporating with the rising temperature. "Maybe we should go outside."

We retreated to the back yard, but there wasn't a whisper of air outside either. We sat still, sapped of energy, drinking glasses of lemonade while we waited for the power to be restored. Kelly flattened herself under my patio chair, panting heavily. A bat fluttered overhead.

After nearly an hour, desperation for something to do set in. I thought of the games we used to play to amuse the kids on trips.

"I packed Grandmother's suitcase," I began, "and in it I put an armadillo."

I turned to Mike, who, according to the game

rules had to add an item that began with the next letter of the alphabet.

He must have been desperate, too. "I packed Grandmother's suitcase and in it I put an armadillo and … a banana."

Andy was quiet. I could imagine his thought process. No computer, no TV. The lemonade. Now word games. *So uncool.* I opened my mouth to take the next turn so the game would keep moving.

But Andy's deep voice came first. "I packed … an armadillo, a banana … and … cotton sheets."

We completed the suitcase game all the way through zooplankton, but no one was up for round two. The power remained out at midnight. We could only think about how uncomfortable we felt. The heavy air made sleeping out of the question.

Kelly sprawled by the front door, sides heaving. "She's not handling the heat so well." I said.

"Let's go out to the van," Mike suggested. I grabbed a pillow off the couch. Andy hitched the leash to Kelly's collar. We all climbed into the van in the driveway, as Mike turned the key and cranked up the air conditioner. It didn't matter how much gas we wasted, as long as the cool air kept gushing from the vents.

Now at least we felt more comfortable. We listened to the radio and took turns dozing. Why hadn't we thought to bring some snacks along? Rubbing my rumbling stomach, I worried about those last few pounds and squirmed on the narrow car seat. I glanced toward the house, hoping to see a sign of power restoration.

Nothing.

Time dragged. Someone snored. This won't be forever, I thought, my eyelids heavy. The lights will come back on. We'll make it through.

My hand rested on Kelly's soft neck. Of course we'd get through. We always did. And if my diet was hitting a rough patch right now, I'd get through that, too. That's the thing about patches, they're just a piece of a larger picture. The healthy habits I'd been learning were what needed to continue. They would stay with me, a change for life. And when things went astray, I just had to be patient, adjust, and find my way out. I'd get through.

Around five the next morning our house suddenly lit up like a shining star. We stumbled inside and fell into bed.

The dog's dinner

Dog movies make me cry. *Old Yeller* was particularlay traumatic in this respect. How could anyone get through that film without weeping like a heartbroken teenager? Some dog movies make me cry because the faithful old dog dies, but I cry just as readily at the happy endings.

When I was a teen I watched a Walt Disney movie, *The Incredible Journey*, one Sunday night while babysitting. The film's three heroes – a Labrador Retriever, an English Bull Terrier, and a Siamese cat – traveled 250 miles through wilderness and treacherous terrain to reunite with their family. The ending – one of the happiest I'd ever seen – left me bawling and blubbering so much that when the parents of my charges returned, they felt sure something awful had happened, and raced around the house searching for signs of a fire or blood. It was some time before I could control myself enough to tell them that the kids were fine and sound asleep!

When we were dating in college, Mike and I attended a showing of Disney's *The Fox and the Hound*. I can't say for sure whether I knew Mike was The One then, but I sure couldn't imagine another guy who'd sit with me in a theater and hold my hand while I teared up over hunting dog Copper realizing he wasn't allowed to remain friends with his red fox pal. Maybe Mike felt it, too. I doubt we will ever outgrow Disney movies.

The parts of any animal movie I don't enjoy are those where there's danger: the snapping bear traps, threatening avalanches and rushing rivers, the porcupines, pack of wolves, snakes, the hunters, even nasty cartoon villains.

Kelly and I encountered a few real-life Cruella De Vils on our walks. For example, some parents tugged their toddlers out of our path. Now, I agree it's never a good idea to let children run up to just any and every dog in the street; we had our share of aggressive dogs in the neighborhood, but these parents never even asked if Kelly was friendly. Wasn't this a sure way to teach children to fear all dogs? I wished I could show them that, under proper circumstances, dogs could be approached and patted and loved, and not feared. No child should miss out on a relationship with a pet, no matter how brief.

Then there were the grouchy homeowners who shooed us away if we just stepped foot on their front lawn. I always carried little plastic bags, and picked up after Kelly. That's just common courtesy.

I was committed to walking because we both needed and, for the most part, enjoyed the exercise, which had contributed to our weight losses. But each trip out, I stayed aware. To me, there was potential for a walk to be as dangerous as those survival scenes in the Disney animal movies.

One late August day Kelly and I ventured out. The weather was perfect; crisp, promising fall. My energy level was up. Kelly's tail flew, and she pranced like a show horse. An ideal day. As was my habit, I scanned up and down the street, on the alert for any loose dogs. If I saw a dog who didn't look particularly friendly, I changed direction, but sometimes it wasn't possible to avoid the dog. A few weeks earlier, a Siberian Husky darted out of its yard and ran at us. I pulled Kelly in the other direction, but it was too late. She saw the dog and lunged toward it.

I was surprised by what happened then. Kelly didn't growl, and her hair stayed flat on her back and neck, unlike other times when every little hair stood to attention. The other dog calmly greeted her. They circled each other, sniffing, and possibly even smiling. It must have been a love connection.

Another time we met a Golden Retriever standing beside her owner in a driveway. The beautiful dog, named Beast(!), turned out to be a gentle soul who played with Kelly on a number of occasions.

I never knew, though, when Kelly was going to start a fight. I couldn't shake this thought when I noticed a burly dog tied to a neighbor's porch railing, large muscles rippling under buff fur. The houses in this section of town stood close to the road, and the dog was sprawled right in the middle of the sidewalk. Nice or not, no way was I going to tempt fate by walking Kelly under this dog's nose. I took one look at the dog and promptly crossed the street.

A large woman came out of her house, wearing a black t-shirt emblazoned with a picture of a skull. This was not a good sign.

"What's the matter with you?" she yelled at me.

"Me?" I mouthed from the other side of the street.

"My baby's not gonna hurt anyone. She's tied up."

It could have been that the woman was just trying to reassure me, but her words were spat out, clearly as accusations, not comfort. She crossed her arms defiantly. "You don't gotta cross the road."

The dog may have been harmless, but now I wasn't sure about the woman. What if she came after us? "It's mine," I said quickly. "*My* dog doesn't like other dogs." I quickened our pace.

"You're a crazy fool," the woman snorted.

Was I? True, I didn't have the best attitude about strange dogs (or strange women). Maybe this woman's misplaced anger, however, was just as wrong as my extreme wariness. Maybe walks didn't have to be so stressful.

Still, we nearly ran the next block. That was enough exercise for one day.

That night Mike surprised me by suggesting we go out to dinner. "How about a date night?"

"Date? We haven't had a date in years."

"Well, the kids aren't kids anymore. Just you and me tonight. Want to go out to dinner?"

"Hmmm, so this is how it's going to be? I like it." Cooking topped my least favorite chore list, and cooking on a diet could be tedious. The same old grilled chicken and salads. "How about we eat anything we want, too!"

"A cheat night?" he asked.

"Italian!" I suggested.

Our first official cheat night began. To be sure, other times we'd cheated, sneaked, slipped, fallen off the wagon, whatever you want to call it, but this time we had planned and approved the event, and I could barely contain my excitement.

We sat together at a cozy white-clothed table in the corner of our neighborhood Italian eatery. I loved the atmosphere, the food, and the money-saving coupon I'd clipped. What more could I want?

Although all diets were off for the night, we eschewed the proffered wine in favor of diet soda. We liked what we liked. A candle flickered between us, illuminating Mike's soft eyes. I wore

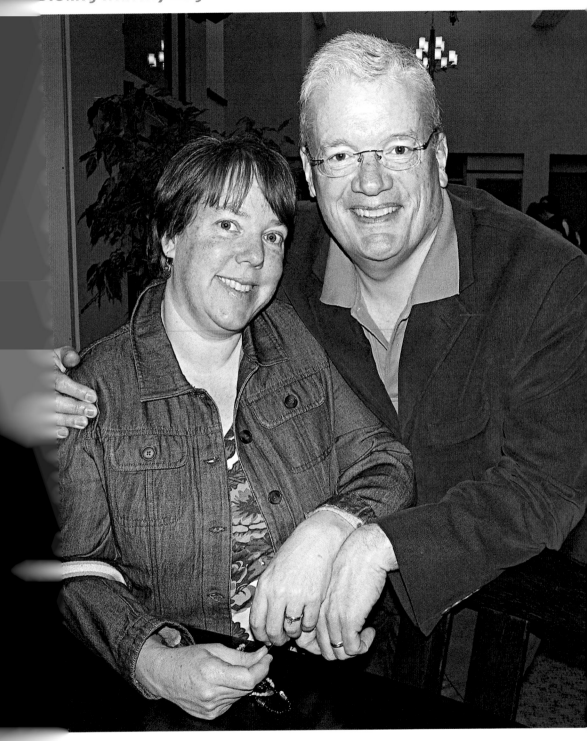

One benefit of the empty nest: more together-time for Mike and me.

my black dress with the v-neckline and high heeled sandals, and had even taken the time to apply blush and mascara. I felt like a grown up. More than that, a woman. For the first time in a long while, I realized I was actually somebody apart from the kids' mom. I was also Mike's wife.

We talked about things – real things like current events, and books and music. We talked about each other. I hadn't realized his work had been so stressful lately, and that somehow he'd contracted poison ivy on his wrist. He listened to me. We didn't try to fix each other, we just shared. I reached over and held his hand. Our feet touched under the table.

The waiter delivered large plates and set them before us. Mike had ordered a Tuscan steak, with potatoes and grilled veggies. I had my favorite: a steaming platter of spaghetti and meatballs. The degree of joy I felt just looking at

that serving of pasta was almost indecent, but I didn't care.

We'd already eaten the crisp salad and warm breadsticks, but now felt ravenous again for our main courses. I twisted my fork in the spaghetti.

"Want to try?" Mike offered me a bite of steak.

"Mmmm." I hadn't tasted steak in nearly a year.

I offered Mike a taste of my dinner. It turned out we were sharing something a heck of a lot deeper than pasta. The mood was light and easy and I felt in love again, like when we were very young. "Here," I used my fork to push a meatball toward him and looked at him with what I hoped were puppy dog eyes.

"Why are you grinning?" he asked.

I nudged the meatball. "It's just like *Lady and the Tramp*," I said.

Every dog has her day

Kelly sprawled on the couch, her paws tucked under her chin, her eyes softly closed. Moments later she jumped up and sprinted with puppy-like energy around the house and skidded to a stop by my side. I kicked a tennis ball with my toe and she chased after it, ears flopping, tail swooshing. She never tired of having fun. *God, I wish I was a dog.*

I sat behind the stacks of papers on my desk, organizing them into manageable piles. I picked up a paper in the first pile and began typing.

Before I finished a page, Kelly trotted back up to me and deposited the tennis ball in my lap. I rolled my chair away from my desk and threw the ball down the hall. She bounced after it playfully. There couldn't be a more agreeable office companion.

With the bright sun shining through the window, I felt energized. I'd been so busy, I hadn't stopped to think about a snack, and now it was lunchtime. Kelly followed me into the kitchen.

The inside of the refrigerator still surprised me every time I opened it. A row of low-fat yogurt cups lined the left side. The crispers brimmed with greens and plump fruit that I actually ate instead of letting turn into moldy science projects. I removed the ingredients for a wholesome sandwich and tossed a baby carrot to Kelly. She caught it in mid-air. She actually enjoyed the crunchy treat now.

Grabbing the multigrain bread from the pantry, I smiled at the pretty glass container of green M&M's: that they'd remained in the jar was another victory.

I sat at the table and chewed my sandwich slowly. Eating felt more relaxed, and so was my work day. No more midday slump.

After I'd been hunched over my desk typing for a while longer, I noticed Kelly sitting in her spot by the front door. She knew what time it was.

"Okay, Kelly," I said, sliding back my chair and grabbing her leash off the hook.

Kelly and I strode briskly along the sidewalk.

"Good afternoon," the older woman who lived on the corner said. I didn't know her name, but she always greeted us, smiling. Nodding at Kelly, she added, "She's full of spit and vinegar."

"Yup, she keeps me going." Kelly wasn't one to let me linger and chat.

Around the corner the usual little girls played outside. "Your dog got a hair cut!" they squealed, running up to pat her. Kelly stopped long enough to kiss their cheeks.

"Her fur's not fat any more?" I asked.

"Noooooo. She's cute!"

We walked long enough to get my heart pumping and cause Kelly to curl up for a deep snooze when we returned.

As I went back to the computer, my Instant Messenger pinged. Judy was checking in.

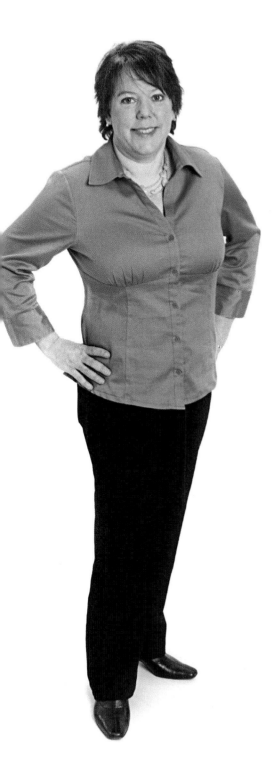

Forty pounds lighter, and feeling good.

"Hey! Just got back from a walk along the trail," she wrote.

"How far?"

"Three miles."

I still couldn't believe how dedicated we'd both become to walking. Not long ago, we were confirmed couch potatoes, exercise not even a sticky note on our day planners. Now, Judy hardly missed an opportunity to walk: in the elementary school gym before teaching; around the block after dinner; with a friend, with her family. I was impressed. She hadn't used her heart attack as an excuse to hold back. I wondered how I would feel about exercising if I'd had a health scare like that. Hers hadn't restricted her at all. "Do you feel vulnerable now, since your heart attack?"

Judy responded right away. "No! Never when I'm exercising. At my physical, all my labs were excellent, my EKG is fine, so I'm not worried."

"Good!" It was wonderful that she felt so strong. Good lab results were reasurring. At my recent check-up, tests showed my cholesterol and sugar levels had improved, too.

"The only time I've felt scared is when I'm stressed. Like the other week I went to the mall and it was really busy, and I felt sort of nauseous and exhausted afterward. That concerned me."

"Were you okay?"

"Yes, but I have to remember to keep my stress under control."

Stress. I felt it, too. We all did at times. It had contributed to my overeating, for sure. When I felt worried I still wanted to grab a snack, and sometimes I did. Other times I practiced new ways to handle stress. The day before, when my computer crashed while I was on deadline, I walked away for a few minutes and took Kelly into the back yard to play. When we came back inside, I was able to deal with the crash more positively.

Dieting with my dog

"How are you doing?" Judy asked. "You've lost forty pounds now. That's quite an accomplishment."

"It's still hard to believe. But at last it's feeling like a habit. I have more confidence, too. I never knew that would happen."

"Me, too! I can get out and walk farther than I ever thought I could. I'm lucky. No more aches and pains. The heart attack wasn't good, but in ways it saved my life. I'm just grateful. I have a lot to be thankful for."

I typed back to her a simple truth: "You inspired me again."

Saturday morning I zipped upstairs to grab my sneakers. At the top of the stairs I stopped and looked back down – had I really just climbed them so quickly? I remembered the days when each step elicited an ache and a groan. Now, not only was scaling the stairs a breeze, but Mike and I were going to take a hike. On purpose!

I snatched up the running shoes from my closet floor. Sneakers of that sort had been missing from my wardrobe for years. Most often I'd simply worn my fuzzy slippers, soft and comfortable. When Mike and I went out, I stepped into clunky clogs or casual mocs, never giving much thought to my image.

After Kate and I went shopping for nice clothes, however, it was fun to take care with my presentation. I'd button up a nice striped blouse. Or fasten pretty sandals. I'd add a necklace. Even if no one else saw me, why not look good for myself? And for Mike. When he came home from work, would he rather be greeted by a wife in slippers and baggy sweats, or one who looked like she cared about herself? I tied my sneakers and pulled a little red short-sleeved shirt over my tank top. Now, outfitted for a hike in the woods, I was dressed better than I had on a good day previously.

Mike and I had never been hiking anywhere before. We got the idea, though, when our walk around the neighborhood became mundane. Never one for challenges before, I surprised even myself by entertaining the idea of something more vigorous.

"What do you think of this?" I'd asked, showing Mike the front page of the newspaper. The story featured popular hiking trails in the nearby countryside. Photographs showed woodsy settings, and a path that opened to a sweeping vista of distant farmland and brilliant blue skies. I didn't relish venturing out into a forest where there might be snakes, bears or who knows what, but if we stuck to the well-traveled trails, there shouldn't be much to worry about. Besides, the views were enticing.

The location was only a half hour from our home, yet we'd never been there before. "We don't have anything going on this weekend …" I'd said, my voice rising guardedly.

Mike, Kelly and I rode out to the trailhead that Saturday morning, earlier than I usually got out of bed. The freshly-dawning day unfurled with a gentle mist rising from the dewy grass. I jumped out of the van with Kelly on the leash. Mike slung a small day pack over his shoulder.

We followed a narrow trail with, in some places, steep drop-offs. "I'm not going to step foot beyond this path," I said.

"Or let go of Kelly." Mike looked down. "She'd be over the edge."

I hoped Kelly wouldn't pull me off the trail. Looking down the path, for a moment I wondered if I'd be able to make it all the way. And then I worried Kelly would tire before we were done. I could just imagine trying to carry her back while managing my own weary body. At home she trotted easily around the block, but we'd never ventured much farther.

Although we hadn't tested her endurance, her new fitness regimen would certainly help with the trek, I reassured myself. At Kelly's last check-up, Dr Dietrich pointed out that she had stronger respiration and better muscle tone.

When Kelly stepped up onto the scale we all cheered; she'd lost six pounds! That was 15

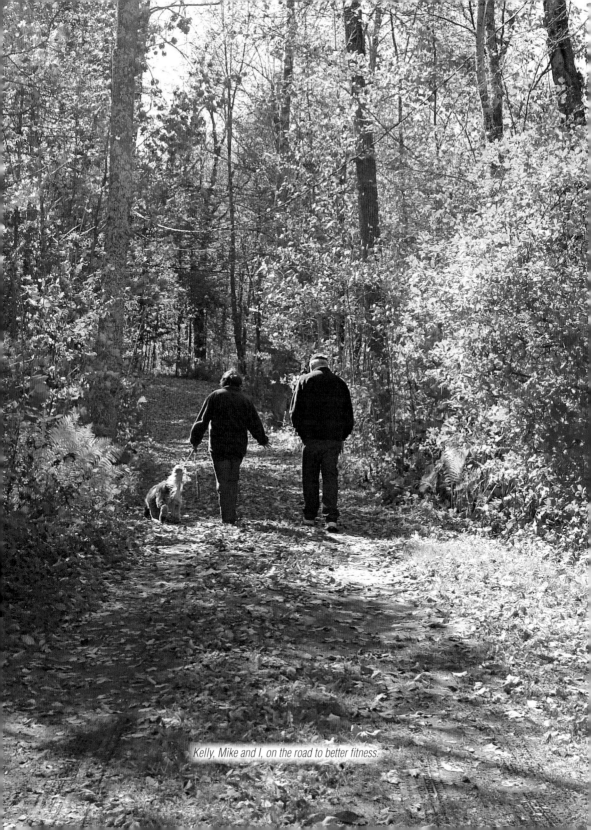

Kelly, Mike and I, on the road to better fitness.

Dieting with my dog

per cent of her body weight. "Perfect!" our vet announced.

Kelly even *looked* stronger as she sniffed along the trail slightly ahead of me. Her back end narrowed proportionately, her sides followed a slimming line beneath her hair. And she moved without a trace of her former waddle.

"Look at this," Mike said at one point, indicating thick limestone formations in a cliff near the side of the trail.

"All those layers," I said, "eroded through the years, all the pretty patterns showing what they've been through."

"It took a lot of time," Mike said, "to make all those stripes."

"Yeah, but it was worth it." I ran my hand along the textured stone as we continued along the trail. So far, Kelly was managing the walk easily. And so was I. My legs felt strong, supporting me along the rocky pathway as I climbed. A balcony of branches covered the trail in some places. "Like walking through a tunnel," I said, actually able to walk *and* talk without panting out each word. I felt my heart pumping, but in a good way; strong and steady. Since my doctor had taken me off my blood pressure medication, I'd maintained normal readings.

"Keep it up," my doctor had said. The worrisome load of concerns about my health that I'd carried for so long was lightening.

Near the end of the hike the path steepened and the exertion became more strenuous, but I pushed myself further. A little further.

"Here we are," Mike said as he reached the clearing. I arrived right after him, with Kelly at my side. She plopped down at our feet, tongue lolling.

"We made it!" I leaned against a rock and took a deep breath. Every shade of lush and abundant green God created spread before me. Dark forest green. Emerald green. A patch of yellow-green. The praise-inspiring green of living and growing things. We were surrounded by a peacefulness resulting from the work of the master artist who'd painted that vista.

"I'm going to rest and enjoy it." I drank from my water bottle. Mike took a portable bowl from the pack and filled it with water for Kelly. We sat alongside the trail and nibbled almonds and apples slices.

"You know," I said, "I wasn't sure I could do it. Even when I was younger I thought this – hiking, healthy stuff – was for other people. It's so different from what I'm used to … and you know how I don't like change."

Mike smiled at me. "But do you now?"

I looked out over the landscape and felt the liberating openness of the great outdoors. "Well," I said. "Maybe not. But yeah, maybe sometimes."

On the way back down we passed a small waterfall. The narrow cascade splashed and disappeared into an underground stream. We stopped and watched the sun sparkle off the spray and dance above the rocks below.

"What a nice day," I said as we drove home. Kelly curled contentedly on the back seat, secured by a comfy harness that kept her safely in place.

"You know, we'll have time to do more things like this together, now that the kids are grown up." Mike said.

"No more worrying about their schedules," I added. "Or parent-teacher conferences, meetings, baseball games."

"No driving them around to school, practice, friends' houses …"

"… or sitting home while they borrow the car."

"Sitting home and worrying," Mike added.

"Yeah, when Andy goes off to college I won't know what he's doing, so I won't have to worry about it."

"Instead you can spend your time worrying about me," Mike teased.

"Or giving you a little attention." I pecked his cheek as he stopped for the light.

"Woohoo!" he said. "This empty nest might just have a silver lining!"

It's a dog's life!

The room consisted of cement block walls, furnished with two narrow beds, two desks and two closets. A roommate had moved in earlier, so one half of the area was cluttered with clothes, towels, packages of microwavable noodles, and even a 32-inch flat screen LCD TV.

Mike, Andy and I stood in the tiny space, surrounded by boxes and duffle bags, baseball equipment, a set of weights, and enough snacks and sports drinks to get through the entire four years.

"This is it," Mike said, clapping Andy on the back proudly.

Yes. This was it; the moment I'd been dreading all summer. My youngest was officially on his own. My job at home was downsized.

I fiddled with the dangling strings that held the window shades. *Don't cry. Andy will be embarrassed.*

No one knew what to do. I opened a box and began to unpack.

"I'll figure all that stuff out later, Mom," Andy said softly.

"I could just hang up your clothes."

"I can do it."

"Stack your books?"

"That's okay."

"How about I make your bed?"

Andy gave in. "Sure, Mom." Mike gave me a look – I'd gone too far, but it was too late now. I unpacked the navy cotton sheets, furled out the folds and smoothed the layers over the thin mattress.

"I think your head should go on this end, don't you?" I suggested, so happy to feel useful that I didn't stop to wait for Andy's response.

Before parting, we strolled around campus. The autumn air smelled crisp and new with the promise of changing seasons. Old stone buildings covered in ivy graced the corners of a leafy quad. Backpack-toting students walked criss-crossy paths in comfortable clusters. I felt their energy. Although I'd fought the idea for so long, I could imagine Andy here. He was capable and mature. This was a great opportunity and he was ready. Maybe we were both ready.

We returned to the parking lot. I wasn't sure Andy had everything he needed, or if I'd told him everything I'd wanted, but the time had come.

"Bye, Mom," he said, giving me a kiss. Right there. In front of everyone. Mike and Andy hugged goodbye. We got in the car and I watched Andy through the rear view mirror until we turned the corner.

At home, I walked in the door. Kelly greeted me. It might have been my imagination, but she seemed to wonder why Andy wasn't with us.

I looked around. This was it. No kids at home. The empty nest.

Dieting with my dog

Look at us now!

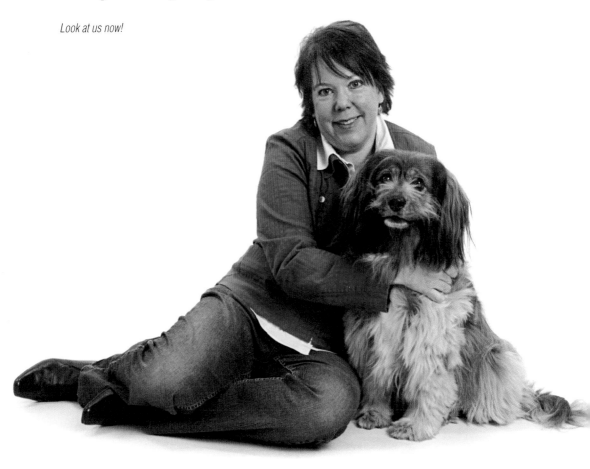

Before dinner, Mike and I took Kelly for a walk. She knew the route well and led the way. A car stopped at the corner and a little girl leaned her head out the open passenger window. "Hi, Kelly!" she shouted. I waved back.

"She's a celebrity," Mike said.

"The little kids like to play with her." As we got out the house and walked more, the neighborhood kids came to expect a visit. Kelly, who could tug on the leash impatiently when she really wanted, knew to stand still and wait for them to finish fussing over her. Just like she seemed to know what I needed, too. At home she still lay by my side as I worked, but also nudged me to get up and get active, too. The empty nest wouldn't be quite so empty with Kelly around. She was my little girl, though I no longer mothered her with treats and table scraps.

"She loves everyone to make a fuss," Mike observed. And that was how I rewarded her now, too, with love and attention.

"What should we do? Want to go out again?" Mike took my hand.

"Let's just stay in. We could even eat dinner in front of a movie. How radical would that be?"

Mike helped me pluck plump red tomatoes

right off the vine from our tiny garden beside the driveway. I set three plates on the table, then remembered and slid one back on the shelf. "I'm still not quite used to this," I said. I wondered what Andy was doing and if he'd had dinner. If he was happy. If he'd made friends. But that was normal. That's what a mother does.

Later, I went upstairs to Kate's room and sat on the edge of her bed. Kelly curled up by my feet. I pressed the speed dial on my cell. "Hey, Mom!" Kate answered. "I'm glad you caught me, we just got back from a long bike ride. So nice out today."

"Here, too," I said. "Almost fall. Soon the leaves will change."

"Same here," she said. "Hey, how'd it go with Andy today?"

"I think he'll do okay."

Kate laughed lightly, knowingly. "And you, Mom?"

"Yeah. I did okay. I'll do fine. He said he'll miss Kelly. But I think he meant he'd miss me."

"Of course," Kate said. "Well, I've got to run, we're going out to dinner with some friends."

"Okay. I miss you."

"Miss you, too, Mom. Oh, and guess what? My friend Sarah just told me she's pregnant! Isn't that great?"

"Oh my, your friends are having babies! Are you getting any ideas?"

"No," Kate laughed again. "Not yet. But when the time is right."

"Of course. Won't that be something!"

"Sure. Can you imagine, some day you'll be a grandma."

I paused, letting that thought sink in.

A grandmother. A new little boy or girl to love. New 'firsts' to experience. Growing up to watch. I'd like that.

"Thanks for talking. I love you."

"Luvya too. Bye Mom."

I smiled as I hung up. Life really was changing. But it was full of beginnings, not endings. I walked across the room and glanced at the near-empty bookshelves. I had books in boxes that would fit there nicely. I moved to the dresser and pulled open a drawer. Only a forgotten pair of socks inside. We didn't really need that piece of furniture anymore. The space would make a good place for my desk, close to the window, where sunlight and a nice breeze would join me while I worked. I could fit my filing cabinet in the other corner. It might work … it might.

Mike appeared in the doorway. "What are you doing in here?" he asked.

"Picturing this room a little different," I replied.

"You mean, a change?" Mike grinned.

I ran my hand across the dresser again. "Could be." No way around it; things changed. The trick was to accept, and even welcome it. Like losing weight, it was a lifetime challenge.

Mike put his arm around my waist and pulled me close. We stood gazing out the window, dusk beginning to settle over the summer sun that still shone through. "Well, this feels different," Mike said. "There's just the two of us here right now."

Kelly rose and wedged herself in-between us. I reached down and stroked her soft neck.

"You mean," I corrected him, smiling, "the three of us."

Appendix

Dog and dog parent weight loss tips from Peggy, Kelly, and friends

Healthy snacks for you and your dog

Six healthy snacks I love
1 almonds (¼ cup)
2 cucumber slices
3 low-fat, high fiber snack bars
4 apples
5 low-cal, fat free hot chocolate
6 strawberries with squirt of light whipped cream

Six healthy snacks Kelly loves
1 baby carrots or carrot coins
2 green beans
3 rice cakes
4 pumpkin
5 banana
6 quality weight-management dog biscuits

Diet tips from Cousin Judy

1 Keep goodies out of easy reach
Put tempting foods high up on a shelf where you can't see –or easily reach – them

2 Don't bring it home
Avoid buying foods you know you can't resist. If someone else in your household eats your favorite cookies or sweets, ask them to hide the tempting treats, and not eat them in front of you

3 Eat more (healthy) snacks
Yes, more! That way you won't be so hungry at mealtimes and overeat, or pick while preparing food. Just make sure your snacks are good for you

4 Make salad preparation easy
To make salads easier to assemble, wash and cut your veggies (or buy them pre-washed and pre-cut) and store in plastic containers in the crisper drawer. When it's time to make your salad, simply pull out the whole drawer and you'll have everything you need in one place

5 Picture the 'before'
Keep a 'before' photograph on the fridge or cupboard door to remind yourself to eat wisely

6 Seek out support
Join a diet and weight loss group, or surround yourself with supportive family and friends

7 Walk, Walk, Walk!
Start slowly, by all means, but get out and do it. It's usually more enjoyable to walk with a friend

8 Stay positive
Keep a list of positive quotes and affirmations,

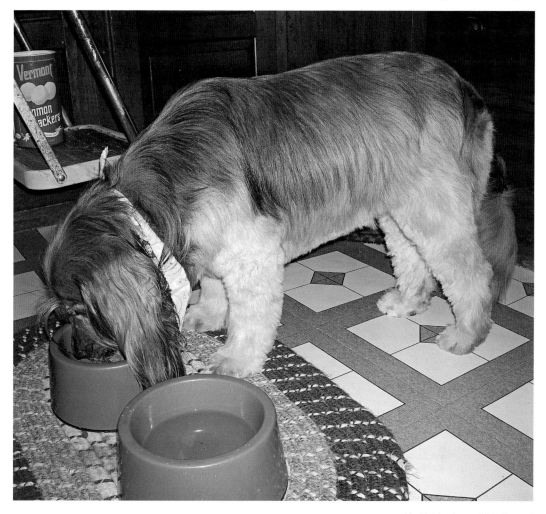

Healthy food can still taste great.

pray, or read from an inspirational book for dieters, like I do

Tips for your dog, from Kelly's vet

Dr Lisa Dietrich, DVM, co-owner of Nassau (NY) Veterinary Clinic, identified Kelly's weight

problem, and started her on the right path to better health. Check out Dr Dietrich's advice for helping your dog lose weight:

1 Arrange for a check-up
Some dogs have medical conditions that cause weight gain, including thyroid problems, early diabetes, and fluid retention from heart disease.

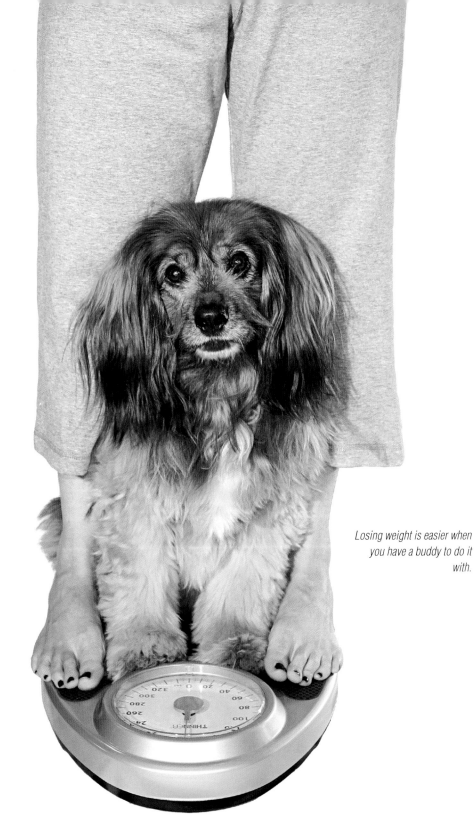

Losing weight is easier when you have a buddy to do it with.

Have your dog checked by a vet to rule out any of these conditions before beginning a diet

2 Get an objective opinion
You might see your dog as a certain size and not realize she's overweight. Asking your vet for an assessment can help put things in perspective

3 Weigh your dog often
Most owners take their dog to the vet about once a year, during which time, weight can be gained without it being obvious. Most vets won't charge for a weight check, and will even help you keep a chart, so a monthly visit is a good idea

4 Measure food
At your dog's check-up, be sure to ask how much food she needs. Then, each mealtime, measure the appropriate amount. A lot of people don't realize they're overfeeding their dog

5 Get physical
Walking your dog, playing, and attending agility classes are all excellent ways to burn calories. For older dogs, keep the walks short and not too strenuous. Your dog might enjoy varied activities and/or scenery

6 Offer low-fat food
Feed your dog a good quality, low-fat dog food. You might want to consider prescription diets available at your vet practice. Also, offer lean treats. Did you know that some over-the-counter dog snacks are as much as 500 calories per treat?

7 Get professional help
Consult a Veterinary Nutritionist if you're struggling. Proper nutrition is not only good for losing weight, but for your dog's overall health

8 Consider medication
If all else fails, ask your vet about weight loss drugs for dogs. They can curb the appetite and help prevent fat from being absorbed. These are best as a short-term solution. You'll still need to learn how to feed and exercise your dog properly so that when she comes off the medication, she won't gain back the weight

Kate's tips for eating out

As a busy professional, my daughter, Kate, often meets her husband after work to grab dinner at a restaurant. Is it possible to make healthy choices when eating out? Here are some of Kate's tips:

1 Be prepared
Visit the restaurant's website before you go out. Search through the menu and plan what you're going to eat. Many restaurant websites include nutritional information. When I go to the restaurant prepared, I'm more likely to stick to healthy options at ordering time

2 Have a bite before you arrive
Eat something healthy before you leave work or the house so that you're not so hungry at the restaurant

3 Start healthily
At the restaurant, fill up on low-fat soup or salad first. (Make sure you bypass the croutons, cheese, and high fat dressings!)

4 Speak up!
Don't be afraid to ask for what you need. Sauces can be left off or served separately. Entrées can be prepared using white wine instead of butter. Extra vegetables can be substituted for potatoes

5 Divide and conquer
Many restaurants are gracious about letting you share. Once, I asked to share a T-bone steak meal, and was happy to see it arrive on two dishes, each with generous helpings of veggies

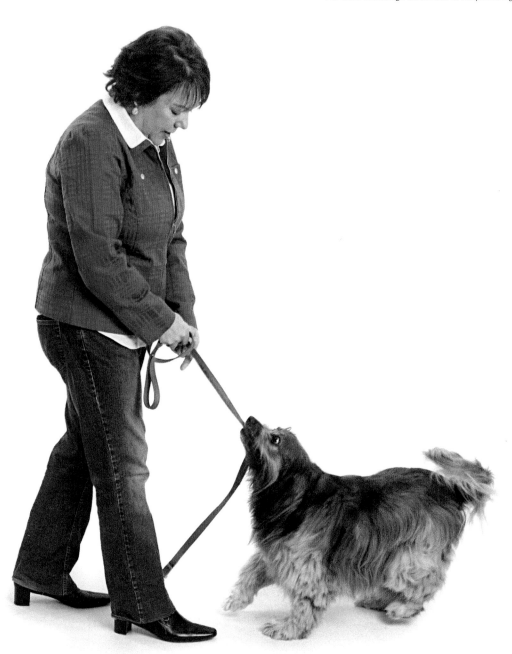

Partners encourage each other to keep moving.

6 Slow down
Eat slowly and enjoy the conversation. Savor every bite. By waiting longer between bites, you'll give your stomach a chance to let you know when it's full

Six ways to exercise together with your dog

1 Take walks
Walk around the block, in a park, or anywhere!

2 Run or jog
Running and jogging is great if you have a dog who can handle the pace, but be careful not to expect too much of her

3 Conduct vigorous training sessions
While reinforcing commands such as 'Come!' and 'Sit!' may not be physically demanding,

energetic play time in-between training is a wonderful reward. And be sure to end the session with a romp around the yard or park

4 Swim
Many dogs love the water and will enjoy swimming with you, or fetching floatable toys. If your dog isn't a strong swimmer, try splashing together along the shoreline

5 Hike
Consider taking your dog along on hikes if she's healthy enough for the activity, and check the regulations for pets on the trails

6 Learn agility
You can construct simple ramps and hurdles yourself, or join an agility club in your community. This activity will keep your dog's mind and body active and fit, and you'll also get plenty of exercise running along the course

Visit Hubble and Hattie on the web: www.hubbleandhattie.com and www.hubbleandhattie.blogspot. com • Details of all books • Special offers • Newsletter • New book news

107

More great books from Hubble and Hattie!

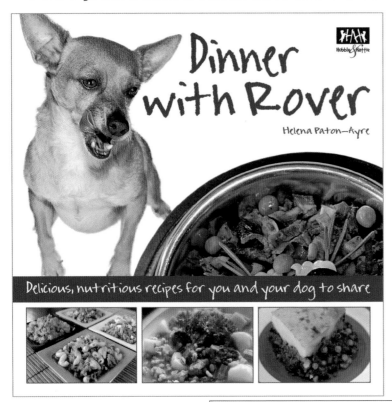

Share breakfast, dinner or lunch with your canine friend: this book is packed with scrumptious recipes that you and your dog will love! Tried and tested by Rover and his friends, and approved by a vet for nutritional value, the recipes in this full-colour book will transform mealtimes!

978-1-845843-13-7
£9.99*

A Dog's Dinner tackles the poisonous pet food problem, and provides forty solutions to it. Special diets are covered for very young and very old canines, sick dogs, and obese dogs, and there are also recipes for treats – because dogs need treats, just like humans.

978-1-845844-05-9
£9.99*

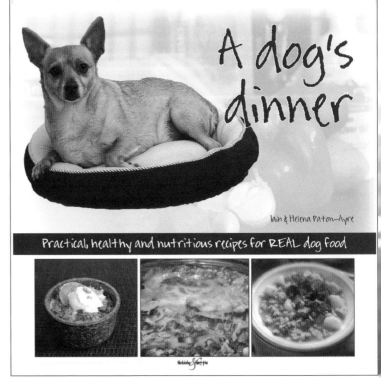

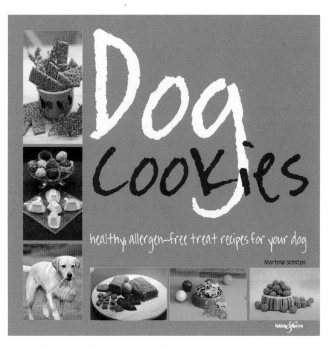

healthy allergen-free treat recipes for your dog

Martina Schöps

- Bake healthy treats for your dog
- Allergen-free dog treats
- Vegetarian dog treats
- Special training treats
- Special ideas for special occasions
  (birthday cake)
- Easy to bake
- Written by an experienced chef and
  dog lover

978-1845843-80-9
£9.99*

Dogs on Wheels – travelling with your canine companion takes a look at you, your family, your vehicle, and most importantly your dog, and tells you how to get the most out of travelling with your four-legged friend – whether for five minutes or five hours.

978-1-845843-79-3
£9.99*

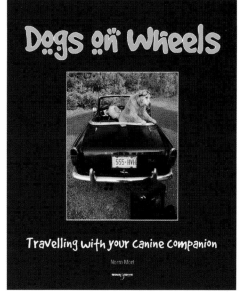

Travelling with your canine companion

Norm Mort

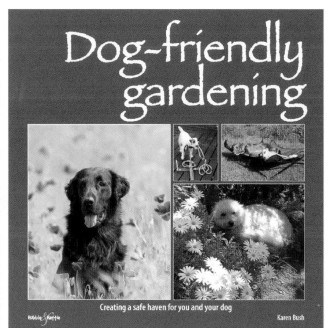

Creating a safe haven for you and your dog

Karen Bush

Even if you're on a budget, with good planning and a little effort you can create an attractive outdoor environment that will actively enhance your relationship with your dog; a place where you can enjoy playing and relaxing together.

978-1-845844-10-3
£12.99*

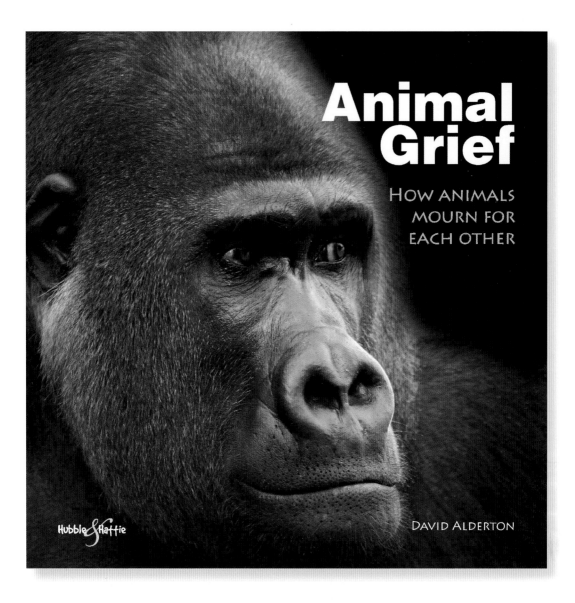

Animal Grief

HOW ANIMALS
MOURN FOR
EACH OTHER

Hubble & Hattie

DAVID ALDERTON

There seems little doubt that animals experience a range of emotions, just as we do; but can they grieve, too ...? This authoritative, rational text is superbly supported by interesting, sensitive photographs, carefully chosen to be reflective of the subject matter.

978-1-845842-88-8
£9.99*

For more info on Hubble and Hattie books, visit www.hubbleandhattie.com; email info@hubbleandhattie.com; tel 44 (0)1305 260068. *Prices subject to change. P&P extra

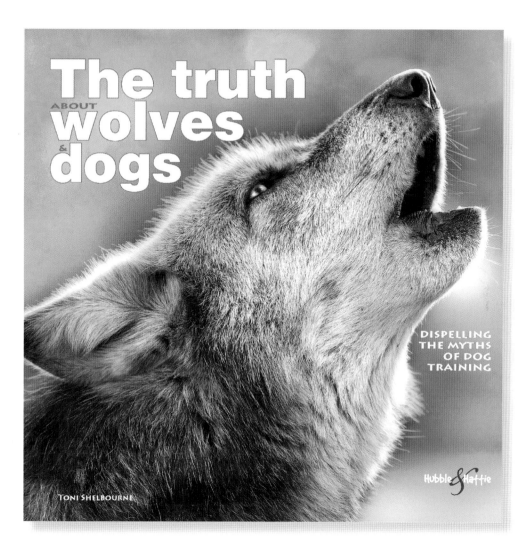

The truth ABOUT wolves & dogs

DISPELLING THE MYTHS OF DOG TRAINING

Hubble & Hattie

TONI SHELBOURNE

A critique of traditional dog training and all the myths surrounding it, prompting the reader to look again at why we do certain things with our dogs. It corrects out-of-date theories on alpha status and dominance training, which have been so prominent over the years, and allows you to consider dog training afresh in order to re-evaluate your relationship with your canine companion, ultimately achieving a partnership based on mutual trust, love and respect.

Your dog will thank you for reading this book.

978-1-845844-27-1
£12.99*

Diet notes

"Peggy Frezon has written a charming and delightful tale. Dieting with my Dog is sweet, funny, inspiring and adorable, just like Peggy and Kelly!" – Julie Klam, bestselling author of You Had Me at Woof: How Dogs Taught Me the Secrets of Happiness

"It only took my reading the first page of Peggy Frezon's book, Dieting with my Dog, and I was hooked! As someone who has dealt with the challenges of weight gain and weight loss all of my life, I was inspired by Peggy's heart-warming story of her journey to make a positive change in her life with the help of her beloved dog, Kelly. Peggy blends humor, candor, and practicality in a wonderful way." – Julie Hadden, from NBC's 'The Biggest Loser' and author of Fat Chance, Losing the Weight, Gaining My Worth

"A quirky and engaging tale of one woman's uncommon solution to a common problem. A moving and instructive celebration of the bond between humans and animals." – Ptolemy Tompkins, author of The Divine Life of Animals, former editor at Guideposts magazine

"Your dog relies on you to keep him healthy. This book is an excellent way to keep the both of you in nice shape; most importantly, by doing it together." – Joel Silverman, Host of Animal Planet's 'Good Dog U' and author of What Color Is Your Dog?

"Dieting with my Dog presents delightful incentives to improve health for people and their canine companions. With the book's rare combination of humor, practicality, and inspiration, readers will become motivated to lose weight and gain a special bond with their dog." – Linda Anderson, co-founder of Angel Animals Network, and co-author of Dogs and the Women Who Love Them, co-author of Animals and the Kids Who Love Them

"Everyone who has ridden the emotional rollercoaster of weight gain and loss, and struggled with the necessary lifestyle changes, will relate to Peggy's battle and eventual triumph over food's controlling grip. Her faithful dog is both an ally and a benefactor of the author's successful journey." – Dawn Kairns, author of MAGGIE: The dog who changed my life

£9.99 UK • $19.95 USA

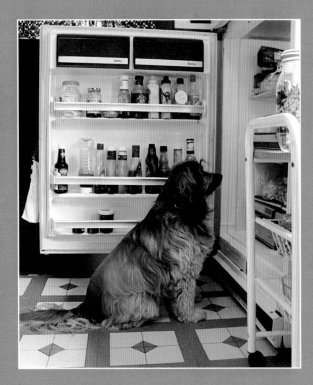

The veterinarian rubbed Kelly's sides for emphasis. "She needs to lose weight. If not …"

Peggy recognized the rundown of serious ailments that followed. It was the same list her doctor had given her.

Dieting with my Dog is the honest and heartfelt story of one overweight woman and her chubby Spaniel, struggling to get fit together. When a busy mom faces the prospect of an empty nest, she turns to her devoted family pet, Kelly – and food. But Kelly soon becomes the motivating factor to facing down the physical and emotional reasons for Peggy's over-eating, and over-feeding her dog. Together, the pair discover that everything's easier with unconditional love.

This book is for anyone who has ever loved an animal – through thick and thin.

ISBN 978-1-845844-06-6

www.hubbleandhattie.com